W9-BEN-622

# Give food a chance:

A new view on childhood eating disorders

Dr. Julie O'Toole

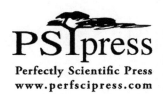

PSIpress

Perfectly Scientific Press
www.perfscipress.com

Perfectly Scientific Press
3754 SE Knight Street
Portland, Oregon 97202

Copyright © 2010 by Perfectly Scientific Press.

All Rights Reserved. No part of this book may be reproduced, used, scanned, or distributed in any printed or electronic form or in any manner without written permission except for brief quotations embodied in critical articles and reviews.

First Perfectly Scientific Press paperback edition: July 2010.

Perfectly Scientific Press paperback ISBN: 1-935638-01-8.

Cover image by Steve Nemirow.
Cover art by Julia Canright.

Visit our website at www.perfscipress.com.

Printed in the United States of America.
9 8 7 6 5 4 3 2 1 0

This book was printed on 15% post-consumer waste paper.

# Preface

I initially wrote this book as a detailed guide for clinicians who care for children with eating disorders. It seemed to me at the time that a technical book written for doctors and nurse practitioners, one readable by an educated lay public, would best serve to spread the message of a new treatment paradigm. On reading it my son Morgan suggested that my audience was all wrong. Write for those who care the most, he told me, write for parents. Parents, he suggested, will care most passionately about the details, will be most motivated to spread the word. Speak to them and they will speak to the doctors. Speak to them and the children will best be served.

# Acknowledgements

There are a lot of people to be grateful to and for when writing a book that basically comprises a whole professional lifetime of work.

Let's start with the personal and most important: I am grateful for my father who modeled the passionate scientist and free-thinker, who believed in me and taught me—a girl child in the 1950's and 60's—that I could be anything I wanted to be and say anything I wanted to say, however irreverent. And for my mother who was the wind beneath both of our wings. Deepest thanks to my husband Steve for naming Kartini Clinic, for helping me understand that it could be done and for just plain making what I do important in our life together. Thanks to my children: My son Morgan who has dedicated his own career to Kartini Clinic's mission and our three girls Sheila, Ariel and Aurora who had to endure things like whole milk and family dinners that none of their friends did. Gratitude to Ben who never understood how his love of science and the natural world inspired me, first as a kid and later as a clinician.

Thanks that can no longer be expressed in person to Frieda Politzer, who taught me to be skeptical of medical practitioners, such as myself, and who suffered much at the hands of psychiatry of the 50's and 60's. A martyr to mother-blaming, she learned to send them all straight to the devil and go her own way. It many ways, because of her courageous example, I could challenge the paradigms of my day.

To the Bundesrepublik Deutschland (Germany) for the great privilege of studying medicine at their invitation and to Professor Johann Buchler (Chemie), Professor Henning Beier (Anatomie), and Professor Aach (Botanik) for giving a young single mother a job. And to those whose friendship there meant everything: Dr Elke Dyck, Dr Inggriani Gandha, Yetty Limoerty-Kremer, Renate Carrell.

And on the professional side I want to thank those who have worked with our kids all these years, feeding, teaching, loving, supporting, inventing and supervising: Shanna Greene, Jade Buchanan, Jayotta Feimoefiafi, Janiece Desocio, Naghmeh Moshtael, Leslie Weisner, Bart Walsh, Megan Lukatch, Beth Sommers, Amy Stauffer, Adela Basayne, Judith Potts, Paul Liebowitz, Jody Dutra, Kimber Khafoury, Kendra Carlton, Sherrill Gandsey and Shari Kerr. And those colleagues to whom I look up: Bryan Lask, Ken Nunn, the late Peter Beumont, Michael Kohn, Iris Litt.

For her courageous, irreverent encouragement and feed-back I thank Laura Lyster-Mensch (Collins) and Jamie Lee Curtis Guest for love, friendship and lightning-like intervention when needed.

A faraway thanks from an invisible disciple to M. Tottori, the originator of "your patients are your teachers." In Honolulu to Dr. John Balfour and Debra Balfour R.N. Thanks to "Dr V." (Emanuel Volgaropoulus) and Bob Worth for opening my eyes to epidemiology and public health.

To the nurses at LBJ Tropical Medical Center in Samoa and the gentle/fierce people they, and I, served.

Many thanks to Richard Crandall, scientific thinker extraordinaire, of PSIpress, for giving this book a chance.

And the kids. I am always grateful for the kids.


Julie O'Toole
Kartini Clinic
Portland, Oregon


June 2010

# Epigraph

O Andi, Molly
now beyond my voice and touch,
my intervention.
Has that siren tongue
whose lashings robbed you of your childhood
finally fallen silent?

# Contents

Preface                                                  i

    Acknowledgements . . . . . . . . . . . . . . . . . . . . . . . . .  i

Epigraph                                               v

Contents                                             vi

**1 Introduction**                                       1

    1.1  Our patients are our teachers . . . . . . . . . . . . . 1

**2 It's a jungle out there**                          9

    2.1  Psychoanalysis . . . . . . . . . . . . . . . . . . 11

    2.2  Hilde Bruch . . . . . . . . . . . . . . . . . . . . 13

    2.3  Feminist theory . . . . . . . . . . . . . . . . . 16

    2.4  Family-blaming theories . . . . . . . . . . . . . 17

    2.5  The media . . . . . . . . . . . . . . . . . . . . 18

    2.6  Current attitudes in adolescent medicine . . . . . . 19

    2.7  Insights from cross-cultural medicine . . . . . . . 20

    2.8  The way we talk . . . . . . . . . . . . . . . . . 23

**3 Why won't my doctor listen?**                27

    3.1  Weight loss and failure to gain weight . . . . . . . . 28

    3.2  Ascertaining the seriousness of weight loss . . . . . 33

    3.3  Common clinical presentations . . . . . . . . . . . 34

    3.4  Common physical manifestations . . . . . . . . . . 41

    3.5  Common laboratory findings . . . . . . . . . . . . 46

| | | |
|---|---|---|
| 3.6 | Other medical disorders presenting as weight loss . | 48 |
| 3.7 | A word about parents . . . . . . . . . . . . . . . | 50 |

**4 Eating disorders of childhood** — **53**

| | | |
|---|---|---|
| 4.1 | Anorexia nervosa . . . . . . . . . . . . . . . . | 56 |
| 4.2 | Bulimia nervosa . . . . . . . . . . . . . . . | 63 |
| 4.3 | Selective eating . . . . . . . . . . . . . . . . | 64 |
| 4.4 | Food phobia/functional dysphagia . . . . . . . . . | 67 |
| 4.5 | Dieting gone awry: Imitative forms . . . . . . . . | 67 |

**5 It is not the parents' fault** — **71**

| | | |
|---|---|---|
| 5.1 | Children do not choose to have anorexia nervosa . . | 75 |

**6 When insurance refuses to pay** — **77**

| | | |
|---|---|---|
| 6.1 | The cost of not referring . . . . . . . . . . . . . | 83 |

**7 Are you telling me it's a brain disorder?** — **91**

| | | |
|---|---|---|
| 7.1 | Neuroimaging . . . . . . . . . . . . . . . . . . | 95 |

**8 What heritability means and what it does not** — **99**

**9 What happens when my child won't eat?** — **109**

| | | |
|---|---|---|
| 9.1 | The Minnesota semi-starvation study . . . . . . . | 109 |

**10 Psychopharmacoloy** — **121**

**11 What is the role of family?** — **135**

| | | |
|---|---|---|
| 11.1 | Unity within the team . . . . . . . . . . . . . | 140 |

**12 What should I expect...?** — **143**

| | | |
|---|---|---|
| 12.1 | Preconsult . . . . . . . . . . . . . . . . . . | 144 |
| 12.2 | Arrival and vitals . . . . . . . . . . . . . . . | 145 |
| 12.3 | Physical exam . . . . . . . . . . . . . . . . . | 147 |

12.4 REDS Interview . . . . . . . . . . . . . . . . . 148

12.5 Parental consult . . . . . . . . . . . . . . . . . 150

12.6 Hospitalization . . . . . . . . . . . . . . . . . 151

12.7 Outpatient follow-up . . . . . . . . . . . . . . . . 153

**13 My child has to go to the hospital?**     **155**

13.1 When to admit . . . . . . . . . . . . . . . . . 156

13.2 The Kartini inpatient eating-disorder unit . . . . . 170

13.3 Medication . . . . . . . . . . . . . . . . . 191

**14 Finally my child is eating. . . what's next?**     **193**

14.1 The day treatment unit . . . . . . . . . . . . . . . 193

14.2 The day treatment program for college-age youth . 207

14.3 Special Issues in the treatment of young adults . . . 211

**15 Is anorexia nervosa chronic or curable?**     **213**

15.1 Maudsley and our family-based outpatient care . . 213

15.2 Is anorexia nervosa a chronic illness? . . . . . . . . 218

15.3 The Kartini clinic meal plan (KCMP) . . . . . . . 223

15.4 Outpatient interventions at the Kartini clinic . . . . 233

15.5 The outpatient course of illness. . . . . . . . . . . 240

15.6 Weight gain and body fat redistribution . . . . . . 244

15.7 Ideal body weight . . . . . . . . . . . . . . . . . 246

15.8 Impediments to healing a child . . . . . . . . . . 251

15.9 No professional anorexics . . . . . . . . . . . . . 262

**16 Food Phobia**     **265**

16.1 Definition . . . . . . . . . . . . . . . . . 266

16.2 Clinical conundrum . . . . . . . . . . . . . . . . 268

16.3 Use of medication . . . . . . . . . . . . . . . . . 269

16.4 Naso-gastric feeds . . . . . . . . . . . . . . . . . 269

16.5 Waiting. . . and waiting . . . . . . . . . . . . . . 270

16.6 Introducing food: Bite, chew, swallow . . . . . . . . 271

16.7 Food phobia case histories . . . . . . . . . . . . . 274

16.8 Discussion . . . . . . . . . . . . . . . . . . . . . . 277

References                                            279

Appendix A:
Rating of eating disorder severity (REDS)             295

Appendix B:
Family history questionnaire for parents              307

Appendix C:
Eating disorder hospital protocol and phases          319

Appendix D:
Eating disorder admission orders                      323

Index                                                 325

# 1 Introduction

## 1.1 Our patients are our teachers

In 1980 I graduated from medical school in Aachen, Germany as an American "foreign student." We had classes in every imaginable subject, the German medical system being extraordinarily thorough: In legal medicine, in forensic medicine, in psychological medicine, and in the more usual areas as well: Pharmacology, neurology, pediatrics, surgery, and so on, covering diseases and conditions common and rare. But no one taught us about anorexia nervosa. We had a classmate who was afflicted. Everyone knew it—it was obvious: She was skeletally thin, the veins in her arms stood out like ropes, her lackluster hair clung thinly to her head, she rode around campus on her bike furiously, exercising, exercising, always exercising, and she was a fantastic student. But she was shunned socially, and the young male medical student she admired was appalled at the deranged appearance she found acceptable.

In 1985 I finished pediatric residency in Honolulu, Hawaii, and returned to the mainland to begin the practice of general pediatrics. As a woman doctor I seemed to pick up several adolescent patients with eating disorders, but I was at a loss to really know how to help them. I listened to them, I pleaded with them, just like everyone else. I referred them to psychiatrists. I rarely heard from or about them again. In 1991 I joined a large pediatric practice in Portland, Oregon, and eventually I established an adolescent medicine practice there. At first there were a few patients with anorexia in this young practice, and gradually there were more. And more. Frustrated colleagues heard I was willing to take on the care of these young sufferers, deemed hopeless by many, and sent them my way.

One of the most challenging cases I ever treated dated from that era: LT, a 14-year-old girl who weighed 68 pounds. I had known of LT; she was a longtime patient of one of my partners, an emaciated, infantilized, difficult child, and I had carefully avoided getting involved. My partner's treatment consisted of reminding her that starving children in Asia would be happy for her share of food, and actually went so far as to recommend a trip to India to her desperate parents. I was sure I had nothing important to offer, and so continued to avoid getting involved. But one evening, when I was the doctor on call, she came in fainting, confused, and with a dangerously low heart rate. Oh, yes, and angry!

Clearly, whoever walks in the door when you are on call is your responsibility. I promptly put her in the hospital. The nurses were appalled both at the hospitalization and the patient. She refused food, of course. She threw food, she cursed the nurses, she had to be physically restrained, we couldn't get her psychiatrist to come and see her in the hospital, she pulled out her IVs, she pulled out her NG tube, spilling her food replacement all over the floor. She howled. This did not make me popular with the hospital staff. I did not know what to do. We had to impose draconian rules on her, which is not the usual *modus operandi* for a pediatrician. We are the good guys. We *like* being the good guys. It was a nightmare, and when she left the hospital, she went right back to starving and exercising, assiduously working off every calorie we had delivered, while continuing with her therapist and nutritionist as before: Arguing, bargaining, and doing whatever the hell she wanted. It was demoralizing, frightening, and discouraging—yet LT was my teacher.

LT, and all the patients whom it has been my privilege to treat after her, were my teachers. Through their suffering and my early abortive attempts at help came the one great insight about their disease that was to change everything for me: Anorexia nervosa is a brain disorder, an organic (biologically based) disease like diabetes or stroke. Neither a lifestyle choice nor a result of poor parenting, it looks organic, it acts organic, it is organic. Furthermore, if anything, it acts most like those great human diseases such as syphilis and tuberculosis whose clinical symptoms, regardless of the patient's age, sex, or nationality, are so characteristic as to be virtually "pathognomonic," a doctor's word for unmistakable. Like rashes, coughs, and bleeding, its manifestations cut right across developmental stages and ages. In most cases, the 10-year-old boys report the same thoughts and concerns as the 19-year-old girls; their delusional beliefs are the same, their core behaviors eerily the same, as if cloned.

This observation flew in the face of accepted psychiatric dogma. Psychiatrists taught that anorexia nervosa was caused by enmeshed mothers and distant fathers. It was conceptualized as a flight from maturity, a manifestation of Western beauty ideals in women, a feminist issue, a family issue, a class issue. Listening to my patients, peering into their families, treating them, this made about as much sense to me as a flat earth or leeches for headache. I found it curious that "scientific" papers were written detailing what the patients said were the "reasons" they had anorexia nervosa. Their medical beliefs were held forth as scientific dogma: "Food was the only thing I could control about my life;" "I didn't want to become my mother;" "I didn't want to become a sexual being." Hadn't anyone read medical history books? Asking patients why they believed they had acquired a disease was a notoriously poor way of determining etiology (cause), and relying on popular opinion was even less reliable. If you had suffered from leprosy in the twelfth century and someone had asked you why you thought you had it, you would almost certainly have replied something to the effect that it was a punishment from God for your sins, and your entire society would have supported you in this belief. Yet it was nonsense. Didn't anyone in psychiatry remember *refrigerator mothers,* the purported cause of autism or *the ulcerogenic personality,* the purported cause of ulcers? That we had been taught in medical school!

I was tremendously helped in the realization of the neurobiological nature of anorexia nervosa by the fact that I was a medical doctor yet not a psychiatrist. I did not have a great backlog of learning to divest myself of. I had been taught virtually nothing about it, which allowed me to see it with open eyes, without preconceived notions. Furthermore, my livelihood did not depend on a series of beliefs about human functioning (such as psychoanalysis) that would have stood in the way of a new treatment paradigm.

As I began to learn about the mechanics of human starvation and re-feeding, I traveled as far as I could to see what was known. Surely I could not be alone in this belief? I went to international eating-disorder conferences throughout the 1990s and made myself mighty unpopular by asserting that, in the twenty-first century, this anorexia, this rare brain disorder, needed reframing. When I spoke up at a conference in London, I was angrily denounced for suggesting we look at anorexia nervosa as a disease not unlike type I (insulin-dependent) diabetes, and as a condition where the patient's underlying genetic vulnerability was acted on by an unknown environmental trigger, initiating a cascade of (predictable) behaviors and symptoms, one that—like type 1 diabetes—could be treated but not eradicated. I pointed out that formerly, type 1 diabetes had also been laid at the feet of mothers feeding their children too much refined sugar. This concept was dismissed firmly by several of the psychologists present. One famous British psychiatrist insisted there was not "one shred of evidence" for a genetic basis to anorexia, and the moderator "reminded" me that it was well known that too much sugar did cause some diabetes!

Lonely in my belief, and with the responsibility for many young patients and their families, I read everything scientific I could get my hands on. I corresponded with overseas physicians and researchers of eating disorders and allied scientific fields. For a while, it appeared the only people who agreed with me were geneticists and veterinarians who studied feeding behavior in mice and rats. I was privileged to find an ear in Roger Cone at Oregon Health Sciences University studying the control of weight in humans and other animals. Working in an atmosphere entirely unencumbered by outdated medical beliefs, and believing only what they could support with data, his team found my approach not odd at all. Genetic vulnerability interacting with environmental "triggers" or agents seemed likely to be the model for most human disease.

In 1998 I went to Stanford University as a visiting scholar to learn what they knew about childhood eating disorders. Iris Litt, a leader in the field of adolescent medicine, acted as my mentor. Stanford was a breath of fresh air and a great opportunity to learn. Although, at the time, my adolescent medicine colleagues there did not share my belief in anorexia nervosa as a brain disorder pure and simple; they had begun to perfect the art of convincing insurance companies that it needed to be treated on a medical (not psychiatric) floor and that no success was possible unless and until weight restoration was given absolute priority. Today this may sound like a given, but throughout the twentieth century and even now, in many places, people who suffer from anorexia nervosa are given years of psychoanalysis or other psychological treatment in the absence of weight restoration. The prognosis with this approach was often poor because physicians had abdicated the field to psychologists and nutritionists who did not focus—no, insist—on the core fact of successful treatment: *Without weight restoration you get nothing.*

In my opinion, bargaining with a brain-starved individual about food and calories and grams of fat has always been worse than useless, especially in children. No doctor would argue with a child about the dose of antibiotics in a case of meningitis, nor surgeon allow a child to tell them how (and if!) a ruptured appendix should be removed, yet respected practitioners withheld lifesaving re-feeding because the child "was not ready to accept it" or was not yet "vested in their own recovery." What nonsense! This disease, this anorexia, with a reported mortality (death) rate of 10%, worse than many diseases considered severe, was allowed to lay waste to a child's body, sometimes for years. Parents read the psychological press about parents being the cause; they were told to "butt out," to leave the topic of food to the psychologist and the patient to deal with. They were told that without psychological acceptance on the patient's part, no amount of "force feeding" would be useful. Desperate, saddened, they watched as their child dwindled away. Pediatricians, also having abandoned the field to psychiatrists and psychologists (between whom they made little distinction), washed their hands of the responsibility for re-feeding and accepted the belief that the parents were the root cause of the disorder.

Armed with the courage my colleagues at Stanford had fostered and the vocal support of my husband Steve, I returned to Portland, left my general pediatric practice and founded the Kartini Clinic for children with all conditions of disordered eating. For the

first few years we focused on building a multidisciplinary team. No
one doctor could do it alone: Diseases of the brain are too severe,
the brain being the core of who we are; too affecting of family,
school, and social functioning for any approach but a holistic one
to work. To keep the focus on weight restoration a physician might
lead the team, but he or she would need to be "first among equals"
as mental health providers and others were added.

At first we focused on inpatient medical stabilization, as the
adolescent-medicine physicians at Stanford had done, followed by
outpatient follow-up. After a few years the appalling rate of repeat
hospitalization forced me to devise a step between the hospital and
outpatient follow-up. The first of several intermediary units (Day
Treatment Units) was created and expanded upon. These step-
down units proved a crucial aid in achieving early and lasting
remission in childhood. Later, a unit was added for college-aged
young adults, an often-forgotten treatment group. Meanwhile
data began to pour in from genetics and the basic sciences about
this, and other, brain disorders once thought volitional. Slowly
people at international conferences became less opposed to hearing
about the biology of eating disorders. I met a handful of Australian
adolescent medicine physicians (Michael Kohn and Simon Clarke of
the University of Sydney), PhD nutritionist Jenny Odea also from
the University of Sydney, and—yes—psychiatrists (Sloane Madden
and the late, great Peter Beumont of the University of Sydney)
who were determined to bring the world of eating disorders into
the twenty-first century. Walter Kaye, formerly of the University
of Pittsburgh School of Medicine and currently at U.C. San Diego,
and Cynthia Bulik at the University of North Carolina at Chapel
Hill have led the research vanguard for the genetic basis of eating
disorders in the United States. At the Kartini Clinic we have

begun a collaboration with Dr. Roger Cone and his team to join others in specifically looking for a locus of vulnerability in children.

And then that battered contingency, the parents, began to collaborate in earnest. The more widespread introduction of family-based approaches has helped hold all providers accountable for reviewing older paradigms of etiology and treatment. It is hard to continue to blame the parents when they prove themselves to be the most powerful agents of change on the clinicians' team.

And the patients continue to be our teachers.

# 2 It's a jungle out there

We are surrounded by a jungle of misinformation, and need to get some things right. Anorexia nervosa is not a modern disease. It was probably known to the ancients, although the first organized descriptions left to us come from European literature. In 1720, in the second edition of his work published in English (earlier editions were in Latin), London physician Richard Morton describes two patients with what we now believe to have been anorexia nervosa [82]. This description was made within the context of a book dedicated to the "consumptive" or "wasting" diseases. Any disease where a patient appeared to waste away was reported by physicians as a "consumptive disease." This would have included tuberculosis, diabetes, and many cancers as well as anorexia nervosa (by far the most rare). Physicians of this era can be forgiven if they were not able to distinguish etiology and divide the diseases accordingly—too little was known. The knowledge of the infectious nature of many diseases, of the causes of some cancers (e.g. smoking, pollution), of the pancreatic injury we call diabetes, lay far in the future. The scientific method was not yet in widespread use; Charles Darwin and Alexander Fleming were not yet born. All medicine rested on empiric (experience-based) observations, many of which were astoundingly accurate and insightful. We are not far from this state today when it comes to understanding brain disorders. With the study of schizophrenia, stroke, and Alzheimer's, we have now begun to recognize the biological basis for what formerly appeared to be "just behavioral."

Because tuberculosis was so common a cause of death in Morton's time and was usually heralded by wasting, thinness in women was not considered a good thing. Yet the description of anorexia nervosa from that era differs little from one that might be written today. In 1684 Dr. Morton was called to treat an 18-year-old girl, "Mrs. Duke's daughter," who "fell into a total suppression of her monthly courses from a multitude of cares and passions of her mind." He thought she had left herself open to this wasting condition for "she was wont by her studying at night, and continual poring upon books, to expose herself both day and night to the injuries of the air, which was at that time extremely cold." He attempted what he could in the form of poultices and herbal medications and diet, though she, "loathing all sorts of medicaments, wholly neglected the care of herself for two full years. Till at last being brought to the last degree of marasmus, or consumption, and thereupon subject to frequent fainting fits..." Morton describes her as "a skeleton only clad with skin," and says, "yet there was no fever, but on the contrary a coldness of the whole body." He declares that anorexia nervosa, "this distemper, as most other nervous distempers, is chronical, but very hard to be cured, unless a physician be called at the beginning of it. At first it flatters and deceives the patient, for which reason it happens for the most part that the physician is consulted too late...." Indeed, his young patient did not respond to treatment, became ever more wasted, and died "of a fainting fit" [82].

The second patient Morton tells us about was a 16-year-old boy (it certainly was not fashionable for males to be thin!) The boy, the son of a reverend, "fell gradually into a total want of appetite, occasioned by his studying too hard..." When the boy did not respond to the doctor's poultices and medications, he was advised to quit his studies and retreat to the countryside to breathe fresh air, ride horses, and drink milk, especially, Morton claimed, asses' milk. I hardly need to point out that this would have been full fat milk, and I was actually able to find out that asses' milk is quite a good source of linoleic and linolenic fatty acids [102]. The boy did, in fact, improve, though Morton was guarded about his long-term cure, as he was never able to fully restore his weight.

## 2.1  Psychoanalysis

Sigmund Freud was born in 1856 in Freiburg, but his family later moved to Vienna. Initially inspired by one of the greatest of all thinkers, Charles Darwin, Freud decided to study science. He claimed reading Goethe's work *On Nature* had directed him toward medicine. He was a talented student, an independent thinker, and a strong student of neurology. His feet were firmly planted in the biology of the brain itself, but what he is remembered for is perhaps more closely related to Goethe than Darwin. Indeed, in his first lecture in the United States, delivered at Clark University in Worcester, Massachusetts in 1909 on the "Origin and Development of Psychoanalysis," while explaining the work with hypnosis pioneered by his early colleague Dr. Josef Breuer with a patient suffering from hysterical paralysis, Freud said: "I have noticed to my considerable satisfaction that the majority of my hearers do not belong to the medical profession. Now do not fear that a medical education is necessary to follow what I have to say. We shall now accompany the doctors a little way, but soon we shall take leave of them..."

He took leave of them indeed, and although some of Freud's theories may have crippled clinical insight into eating disorders for the better part of a century, it was not because he was not a great thinker. His theories on mental disorders and human motivation (not to mention war, death, and civilization) were based on observing patients in his own practice and thinking about them. Later, however, his theories were enshrined as dogma in psychiatric textbooks, long after their useful application to the practice of medicine became dated. Yet there are still practitioners of psychoanalysis in the twenty-first century who treat patients suffering from anorexia nervosa with talk sessions stretching out over years, exploring unresolved unconscious conflicts that are supposed to be causing the anorexia, while the patient remains at a dangerously low weight and the family is advised to disengage, despite obvious medical impairment. We modern non-psychiatric physicians, who understand little of Freud's or any other type of psychoanalysis, have been only too happy to abdicate the field to these practitioners when we felt unable to manage a young patient who appeared not to "want" to get well. Suddenly the very doctors who relish a clinical enigma or a "challenging case" and who are taught to do truly difficult things such spinal taps in a newborn, feel helpless. Physicians who would laugh at the idea of discussing the dose of an antibiotic with a child who has meningitis, suddenly decide that a patient with anorexia nervosa cannot be re-fed without her permission and must be consulted about how many calories and grams of fat she is willing to consume. Thus, the brain ceased to be the most complex and interesting organ in the body and became a black box, one to be opened by priests or therapists only.

"We must recollect that all of our provisional ideas in psychology will presumably one day be based on an organic substructure," Freud reminds us in his *On Narcissism* [31]. Ironically that may well be the most modern word on the subject.

## 2.2　Hilde Bruch

In the 1930s, a young Jewish woman named Hilde Bruch living on the border of Holland and Germany defied tradition for women her age and went to medical school. Alone in her family to recognize the danger to Jews that Hitler posed, she left Europe for London and then for the United States. She became a pediatrician, with a strong background in physiology [9]. She lost most of her family in the Holocaust and, according to the biographical information gleaned from her papers at the Texas Medical Center, became clinically depressed. This illness, along with her belief that obese children were fat for psychological reasons, prompted her interest in psychiatry. She actually became a psychiatrist whose primary research interest was obesity. This work with obese children led her to another group of patients with weight control issues: Sufferers of anorexia nervosa. Dr. Bruch is perhaps one of the best-known and most quoted sources on anorexia nervosa, and although (in my opinion) she made some astute observations, she did also refer to these patients as "individuals who misuse the eating function in their efforts to solve or camouflage the problems of living that to them otherwise appear insoluble" [10]. This characterization has stuck like glue to professional discussions of anorexia nervosa, to the detriment, I believe, of really understanding the brain science at its core. I discuss this in a moment when we think about the way we talk.

We are told that upon accepting a position in the department of psychiatry at Baylor, Bruch bought a Rolls Royce (!) and moved to Texas to begin her private practice [113]. In her papers from this era we read that she observed anorexia nervosa to be a disorder of the affluent. Could hers have been a biased sample? It seems likely that the patients who appeared in the private practice of a Rolls Royce-driving psychiatrist would, indeed, have been more affluent than not, representing a true selection bias. Although this observation of Bruch's has not been confirmed by contemporary clinical experience or research, it lingers as a truism in the lay press and has proven amazingly difficult to dislodge. Rachel Bryant-Waugh and Jacqueline Doyle in their chapter on the epidemiology of anorexia nervosa in *Anorexia Nervosa and Related Eating Disorders in Childhood and Adolescence* note that "a number of studies of non-clinical populations have failed to show that social class is a significant risk factor in the development of eating disorders" [90].

Looking back over the history of science and medicine we can see that two things happen frequently when all observations are empirical or based on clinical observation alone: 1) Personal beliefs and prejudices of outstanding (or at least vocal) practitioners begin as "theory," then go unchallenged as "fact," and 2) trends in small populations are extrapolated to everyone without consideration for how such a small sample size might be skewed by circumstances. If, for example, you were Irish and had a practice devoted to a rare condition at a time when few other people were studying this condition, and further, you had a crucifix on your office wall and were well known in the local parish of mostly Irish immigrants (as was once common), you can imagine that your patients might be disproportionately Catholic. If you then wrote a book reporting all the cases you had treated, people might be forgiven for thinking this disease more common among Irish Catholics. Say the disease was a mental disease, and your book postulated that its cause had something to do with "Catholic guilt." Then when a young Jewish doctor read your book and saw the word *guilt,* she would be looking for guilt whenever she saw a patient with this disease among Jewish patients. Guilt is common among humans, so she would find it. Then she could write a book based on "guilt" and the mental disorders it "causes," referring to your experience. If no one troubled with controlled studies (this often happens with rare diseases), the concept of guilt "causing" this mental disorder could easily become a part of the prevailing dogma. In the same way, early concepts about the causes of mental illness such as "penis envy" or "refrigerator mothers" or "oral impregnation" could go unchallenged by data for many years and become an entrenched part of medical teaching.

Hilde Bruch was not unaware of this tendency in medicine and once noted: "Psychoanalysis played an important role in bringing about a new understanding of psychological factors, but *it presented its principal theoretical assumptions as fixed knowledge,* the way many topics were presented as definite at that time. [Italics are mine.] Investigative focus was on the disturbed eating function, the 'oral' component. Anorexia was viewed as a form of conversion hysteria that symbolically expressed repudiation of sexuality, specifically of 'oral impregnation' fantasies. This view dominated the field during the 1940s and 1950s and has not yet completely departed" [32].

I'll say! As a community practitioner I can tell you that it is not uncommon to give a talk and have either therapists or sufferers express their firm belief that anorexia nervosa (AN) is a repudiation of sexuality or a result of sex abuse, especially forced oral sex or fantasies thereof. Because these things seem to make "intuitive" sense, they are repeated as fact. I have had insurance companies insist that a patient's illness is "obviously" a result of traumatic parenting or a refusal to grow up, i.e. a "control" issue. As recently as 2004 I witnessed a serious discussion between psychiatrists online who referred to a colleague's concept of bulimia nervosa as a patient "regurgitating the mother." It makes a good story, I suppose, but will need to survive the scrutiny of contemporary science.

## 2.3   Feminist theory

In the late decades of the twentieth century, educated women began to think about medical issues affecting women primarily. *Self-help* and *empowerment* became buzzwords. This is not trivial stuff: Women have been, and still are, disenfranchised throughout much of the world; little girls' aspirations are not given the same airing as little boys', their education is curtailed, their careers are limited, and worse, much worse. This is all true, but what does it have to do with anorexia nervosa? Feminist theorists postulate that anorexia nervosa is caused by a fear of fat as an expression of fear of women's power. Susan Bordo, professor of English and women's studies at the University of Kentucky, writes, "female hunger—for public power, for independence, for sexual gratification—[must] be contained, and the public space that women be allowed to take up be circumscribed, limited... On the body of the anorexic woman such rules are grimly and deeply etched" [8].

I find it interesting that in the search for the etiology of a severe medical condition such as anorexia nervosa a professor of English can have such influence and credibility. And why just anorexia? It is hardly the only disease to strike a preponderance of women. Systemic lupus (SLE), a severe auto-immune disorder, is one such disease; about 90% of lupus patients are young women between 15 and 45 [93]. Lupus affects many different organ systems, including the brain. Does that make it a feminist issue? Because lupus presents with a rash, does that make it seem more "medical" than a disease like AN that does not? The discussion raised by feminist theorists is very interesting, but what does it have to do with the sick, terrified 10-year-old boy with anorexia nervosa who lives on an isolated farm? When I look into his eyes, when I hear his concerns (identical to those of older, female patients), I feel anger at theories that trivialize his suffering and try to make it someone's fault, try to make his family feel that, given the right stuff, he could just think his way out of this "cultural box." Mistaking cause and effect or ascribing causal meaning to coinciding events is a common mistake. Because anorexia nervosa is more common among women does not make it a psychosocial disease of women. Sickle cell anemia is much, much more common among African Americans than Caucasian Americans. Does that make it a psychosocial disease? Acute lymphoblastic leukemia is more common among children of upper socioeconomic class [96]. Does that mean its causes are psychosocial?

## 2.4 Family-blaming theories

Authors who claim to see only one type of family or family functioning in "anorexogenic families" have dominated many discussions of the past. Even astute observers such as Salvador Minuchin have left us with the idea that families of anorexic patients are characterized by enmeshment (parental over involvement), over protectiveness, rigidity, and lack of conflict resolution. I have wondered about this for years, interviewing and working with such families. The parents of children with AN who arrive in our clinic are desperate, or they would not be there. When our children are ill, we are not at our best. When we feel blamed or guilty, we are definitely at our worst. I have watched difficult parents transform into reasonable, easy-to-work-with parents as their child got better. Of course, some parents are rigid, as some people are rigid—but these are temperament types, probably powerfully under genetic control. Could rigidity run in families of children with anorexia? Certainly. But I regard this as equivalent to saying high cholesterol runs in such families—an absolutely nonpejorative statement that carries with it not only no blame, but no certain connection to causality. We fight this notion that temperament traits are under genetic control because *we* want to be in control. *We* want to choose to change or not. If the patient cannot control his temperament, then, by implication, neither can the doctor!

Regarding "over protectiveness and enmeshment" (a charge overwhelmingly leveled at mothers), I think we may have the cause and effect mixed up here: I think that mothers have a very fine, instinctive understanding of when their offspring are vulnerable or wounded, often long before it is apparent to others, and that they then draw close. Throughout the animal kingdom the female draws close to her wounded offspring. Saying the mother is "abnormally" close to an ill child, and that this must therefore be the cause of the child's illness, needs, in my view, a hard rethinking.

## 2.5 The media

Now for the media. I feel weary as I write this. Try an experiment: Type "media anorexia nervosa" into a search engine on the Web. I got 338,000 citations. Media coverage of eating disorders is ubiquitous, overwhelming, and—often—unhelpful. There can be no doubt that our Western contemporary society values slenderness, even extreme slenderness, in women, just as it values youthfulness. But I find it trivializing and insulting to our young and very ill patients to imply they are "doing this" to achieve a certain look.

Although we have had children who were home-schooled, lived on a farm, read no magazines, and watched little to no TV develop anorexia nervosa, the majority of our patients are bombarded by the media, just as we all are. To say that the media "causes" eating disorders is a little like saying that breathing does. We all breathe. Yet it is clear that the drive to be terribly thin does immensely complicate efforts at weight restoration. More about that later.

## 2.6   Current attitudes in adolescent medicine

I always liked teenagers and thought them an overlooked and under appreciated class of pediatric patients and I still think so. When I first took my Boards in adolescent medicine I was thrilled to be among doctors who thought so too, especially since a couple of them were my most admired colleagues (and still are). But I was made a little uncomfortable by an attitude that prevailed in adolescent medicine conferences and writings that seemed to me to actually pit adolescents against their parents. Parents were often represented as intrusive, controlling people who were trying to foist outdated moral beliefs onto contemporary adolescents. Teenagers were supposed to make autonomous decisions, they said, not only in the area of reproductive health, but also in the areas of sexually transmitted diseases, substance use and abuse, education, and relationships. The primary relationship was not seen to be between a child and their family, but rather between child and doctor. The doctor routinely—and by design—withheld medical information from parents. It was made very clear to teens that this was their right, the way things should be. Adolescent medicine had adopted what I consider to be one of the most counterproductive remnants of the 20th century, that holiest of holiest: Sacred confidentiality between psychotherapist and patient.

What is wrong with confidentiality, you might ask? Won't people refuse to talk if they aren't assured of it? I don't know about "people," but I know kids will talk, because they want to be heard. Even if they think you might tell their parents, in fact, sometimes because they need you to tell their parents, they will often talk because they want an adult to act like an adult.

In my opinion, to treat therapists, especially psychiatrists (and more recently adolescent medicine doctors) as secular priests whose confidentiality is absolute, even before the law, keeps psychiatric illnesses stigmatized. There are even psychiatric offices where entrance and exit are planned so that no patient could ever be "identified" by anyone else as a person in need of psychiatric or psychological care. In the rest of medicine, even in those sub-specialties which routinely deal with sensitive medical issues such as urology or gynecology, no attempt is made to disguise or conceal the fact that anyone is a patient there. Until we are able to treat brain disorders (psychiatric disorders) as disorders along the same continuum as all medical disorders and treat them with the same respectful confidentiality *but no more* than other illnesses, we will perpetuate the shame.

## 2.7 Insights from cross-cultural medicine

I have had the privilege of practicing medicine and of training to practice medicine in several cross-cultural settings. It changed my life and my perspective on treatment practices. Some of our attitudes and beliefs about eating disorders would benefit from a "cross-cultural" analysis.

My first cross-cultural experience was as a medical student in Germany where there were no other American students. This threw me back on two very different groups to learn from and socialize with: German students and their families and other foreign students, like me.

From the Germans I learned about structure, stability and predictability and their beneficial effects on family life and on children. From them I also learned that meals were not always as I had known them growing up: The main meal of the day could be at noon and be dinner-like in its quality, quantity and family base. "Dinner" (*Abendbrot*) could then be smaller, cold and composed of salads and breads with cheese. Both of these meals could be eaten happily in a family setting without anyone complaining that they interfered with school or sports. Neither sports nor work interfered with the orderliness of family life and mealtimes, as mealtimes were a *priority*. No one challenged this social good. I learned that even a coffee break at work was, or could be, a communal event, where everyone stopped for fifteen minutes, spread a white table cloth, poured good coffee into porcelain cups and took a true social break—even within the hospital. There was no hurried cup of purchased coffee in Styrofoam cups, sipped at a work station. Eating (and drinking) was mindful. The day was paced humanely.

But it was from my Asian fellow-students that I learned the most. For the Asian students who were mostly Chinese-Indonesians, food and meals were of paramount importance no matter how poor we were. Food was always cooked communally and eaten together. Parties were about eating together, not primarily about alcohol. None of them would go to a party without food—what was the point? They taught me to make wonderful meals from cheap ingredients and to stretch them to accommodate one more guest. But they also taught me to think critically about the role of parents in the lives of children. They challenged the Wester belief that teens "need to individuate" from their parents as a priority of late adolescence. They were puzzled by our belief that we needed to break away from our parents, form nuclear families of our own and then "learn to let go" of our own children. It became clear that what I had learned as scientific tenets were just cultural beliefs with no more validity and science behind them than any other cultural practices or beliefs. Asian youth were not ashamed to live with their parents until they married in their late twenties or early thirties. They did not see children or teens—barring tragedy—as existing outside of the context of their extended families. Multi-generational family groups living together was seen as a positive arrangement in the lives of children. Back home, they told me, their parents or uncles and aunts often attended some of the same social events as the youth themselves, without being looked on as spies or unwelcome chaperones, and yet there were very clear intergenerational boundaries.

My next cross-cultural medical experience was in Hawaii, noto-riously a mixed salad of many ethnic groups, most of whom (except for Caucasians from the mainland) are very family-oriented. In the hospital in Honolulu, no local Polynesian child was ever left alone at night. Aunties, uncles, cousins, grandparents, etc. would bring favorite foods and sleep on the floor if necessary. Independence from their families was not the chief goal of growing up. This attitude was even more pronounced in Samoa where I was privileged to work for a short while. There, a relatively culturally intact people still lives in the belief that each are a part of the whole. In Samoa, when a child dies, he or she is buried next to their home, in the "front yard," so as to remain near the family forever.

When I finally returned to the mainland to practice pediatrics and adolescent medicine, I was startled and somewhat saddened to find the emphasis on excluding the parents from treatment, especially for teens. I myself had the experience of taking my oldest daughter to a therapist for some adjustment counseling and being treated, literally, as the checkbook. I brought her to her (very nice) counselor, signed the check, and was never once kept informed about what was being discussed. My role was as the chauffeur and the one who signed the check. I tried not to ask my daughter about her sessions, since the therapist made it clear that therapy was "between them" and I was afraid to be seen as an over-bearing and intrusive parent. I have become even more uncomfortable with this approach to children and teens with the passage of time whether I am the doctor or the parent. In the context of a severe illness, such as an eating disorder, I feel it is even more inappropriate.

Children belong to their parents. With very few exceptions, parents love their own children more than the doctor ever can and are deeply concerned with their welfare. Furthermore, children actually resemble their parents because they are their closest genetic relatives and most often share their family's values. It is far more important that a child share the value systems of his or her family rather than the doctor's.

## 2.8   The way we talk

Now I have begun to feel a little like that famous chef of *Cook's Illustrated* magazine who reports on all the awful ways recipes have been handled by others and who, with experimentation and ceaseless testing, now gives us the one Right Recipe, the Correct Way to Cook. There is no one right recipe in medicine or science. Richard Morton, Hilde Bruch, and Sigmund Freud were not small thinkers nor benighted ignorants; rather they were great thinkers, explorers, and observers. Benighted is when their theories are presented as dogma; benighted is when we do not challenge and rethink what has gone before and what is current today. There are no unassailable ideas in science, no theories so true that they are the one Right Recipe. Even very safe-seeming concepts such as time and gravity get challenged to their core. To stand still intellectually is to accept intellectual extinction. Data trumps theory, data drives or informs theory, and therefore theory must remain in constant motion.[1]

In reviewing the thinking about anorexia nervosa that has gone before our "era of the brain," even though we may repudiate much of it, we are still left with old ways of talking about this brain disorder that carry strong, subliminal subtext messages with them. We should be careful. We can give lip service to the neurobiological nature of eating disorders and still say things like, "We just want to find out why she is doing this;" "What role is this patient's eating disorder fulfilling in her life?;" "She's not ready to give up her eating disorder;" "I think we need to get at the root of why she has anorexia;" "What does her eating disorder *mean*?" and so forth.

How can we be more careful about what we say? Why does it matter?

---

[1]For a review of the slow acceptance of evidence and data-based psychotherapies (such as cognitive-based therapies) in the wider therapeutic and medical communities of today, it is instructive to read an article by Timothy B. Baker et al. See [2].

Try substituting the word *leukemia* for *anorexia* and see if
things seem clearer: "What role is leukemia fulfilling in her life?;"
"She's not ready to give up her leukemia yet;" "I think we need to
get at the root of why she has leukemia;" "What does her leukemia
*mean*?" It sounds ridiculous, and it is. Children and young adults
are very sensitive to subtexts that appear to contradict the primary
text. They hear what sounds like ambivalence. They don't believe
you mean what you say. Perhaps, they think, anorexia nervosa *is*
their fault after all!

What we say matters. It matters a lot.

# 3 Why won't my doctor listen?

Every young pediatrician sees a case of anorexia nervosa in the hospital at least once during his or her training. Perhaps they help take care of the patient, perhaps not. They are usually aware of the patient's emaciation, need for weight gain, and any electrolyte or cardiac problems they may have. These are the kinds of things doctors focus on. These are the kinds of things they *like* to focus on. What they do not like and commonly have no talent for is managing psychological or social symptoms. Doctors often fear that patients with anorexia nervosa have many other psychosocial problems as well; after all, aren't they treated only on psychiatric wards in some institutions? This fear makes patients with anorexia nervosa highly suspect to the general medical team. No one talks about the fact that almost all patients with serious chronic illnesses have multiple psychosocial issues too. Overworked and overwhelmed, for the most part, young doctors in training do what they must in the hospital for these patients and hope (in vain) that they will not have to deal with them once they are out in their own private practice.

Anorexia nervosa is rare enough that it is often a long time before a patient walks in the door of a private general pediatric practice, but almost no one practices for any length of time without encountering an eating-disordered patient.

When eating-disordered patients do present in a general clinic, like all other patients, they have no label defining them as such. Children with anorexia nervosa may present in many different ways, and the astute and conscientious practitioner needs to be aware of them. Once an eating disorder is suspected, they need to know what to do and when to recognize that they, the practitioner, are out of their depth and need to refer this patient to a specialty clinic.

Let's talk about this "early recognition." What are some of the common ways for young patients with anorexia nervosa or other eating disorders of childhood to present, and how can the doctor be fooled? Below is a description written for a doctor or nurse practitioner which an interested parent might find useful to share. Throughout this book the term "doctor" is used as a shorthand to refer to all physicians and nurse practitioners who see and treat children.

# 3.1    Weight loss and failure to gain weight

Weight loss is a tricky subject. Our society is becoming increasingly focused on a reported epidemic of obesity. One of the side effects of this focus is that any weight loss is considered a good thing. But as a clinical practitioner, be careful: Weight loss in childhood is rarely a good thing, even in overweight children. Young animals, including human children, spend their childhood in growth: Somatic (bodily) growth, brain growth, social growth. As a child increases in height, his or her weight must also go up. It never goes down; at least it should not. The *rate* of growth may be uneven, with periods of more rapid growth during infancy and again at puberty, but a growth chart should show a weight and a height curve that goes steadily up, staying more or less along the same percentile after the age of two. It should not go down. Any actual weight loss heralds a problem (not always an eating disorder) until proven otherwise, even in fat children. Unless a practitioner is certain that weight loss in an obese or overweight child is supervised, intended *and monitored*, he or she must begin to take a history including questions such as: "What did you have for breakfast this morning? Last night for dinner?" The answers will need to be corroborated by a parent. Nonspecific questions such as "Do you eat dinner?" will not give the same result as the "pop-quiz" nature of a question like: "What did you eat for lunch *today*?" Even if the doctor is satisfied with the answer, a note needs to go in the chart asking that this child be weighed at all future visits, even for simple things such as earache. At the Kartini Clinic we have seen several boys who were "chubby" adolescents, lost significant weight (because of an undiagnosed eating disorder), and had permanent growth stunting by the time it was detected. The parents were understandably upset by the lack of weight-loss documentation and intervention on the part of their physician.

Fat children get anorexia nervosa, too, and it is not a good trade-off, although people are tempted to think it is. If a fat child is losing weight, ask the same questions that you would of a thin child or one of more average weight. Avoid saying things like, "good for you," or "you look great," until you are certain you understand what is going on. If the child reports cutting out all fat, stopping eating fast food, and increasing exercise, be deeply suspicious, but not negative. Explain that although this sounds like they are taking a laudable interest in good health, it would be a good idea to check their weight again in a month. Chances are they won't resist this, because—eating disordered or not—people are commonly proud of weight loss. This is where the media pressure really plays a role. Children will have absorbed the message "all weight loss is good" loud and clear, and only the doctor will have (or should have) the perspective to be cautious. Parents of fat children are commonly also very enthusiastic about their child's weight loss. Fat children often present to the specialized eating-disorder clinic far sicker and more compromised than children who were not premorbidly fat, because everyone was so busy encouraging their weight loss, they paid no attention to their vitals, especially their heart rate. It often isn't until such a child faints in school that they come to the attention of a specialized eating-disorder clinic.

I want to pause for a moment to discuss my use of the word "fat." This is not a book written for children. This is a chapter on pediatric weight and weight monitoring. No attempt is made to be politically correct or even diplomatic. It is very important to me for practitioners to understand that those patients whom they perceive as "fat" need the same monitoring for eating pathology and weight loss as much thinner patients do. Here, I use the short-hand "fat" rather than words such as "overweight" or "larger" with less punch in order to cut through prejudices that we too harbor in the medical community. I am a vocal advocate of "size acceptance" given the embryonic state of the science of weight regulation in humans, but that is for another discussion.

At the Kartini Clinic, where we speak to and about children, we refer to the patients we see for obesity-related issues as "children of high body weight."

*Failure to gain weight* is a more complex symptom, but not one that should fool a pediatrician or pediatric nurse practitioner, as it is discussed in every pediatric textbook. The curve along which a child grows during the first year or two of life mostly reflects the biological mother's age, parity, and uterine health, and it isn't until after the second year of life that we see a child growing along the percentile that more accurately reflects their own genetic growth potential [60]. Faithfully charting a child's growth on a growth chart is an essential of good pediatric care for many reasons. Over time, a child's growth should move steadily upward, canalized along their own personal percentile. We are often referred prepubertal children whose weight and/or height has not changed for a year or more (average rate of change in height should be about 6-7 cm/year and weight gain of less than 2.2 lbs (1 kg)/year has been cited as being below the 3rd percentile in all growing children) [81].

Most pediatricians would agree that this "failure to gain in height and weight" warrants further examination. In such cases, a thorough food history is much cheaper and faster than a major endocrinological or gastroenterological or cardiac workup. If the answer is in the food intake, you know where to start. If the answer seems less clear-cut than that, one of the other specialty workups may be indicated [60, p. 133-134].

Understanding growth in childhood is essential to knowing how to think about weight loss. As puberty is only loosely correlated with concepts like "adolescence" or "teen years," it is important to understand the relationship of pubertal staging (known by many as Tanner Staging or SMR) to growth in height and weight.

The average caucasian American girl initiates thelarche (breast budding) at about ten to ten and a half years of age, at which point she enters the last great somatic (bodily) growth spurt of her entire life, which will last about two years and will include the onset of menstruation. This means that the average fourteen year old girl is nearly fully grown in height, which obviously means that "failure to gain weight" means something different for an average 11-year-old girl than it does for an average 15-year-old girl who

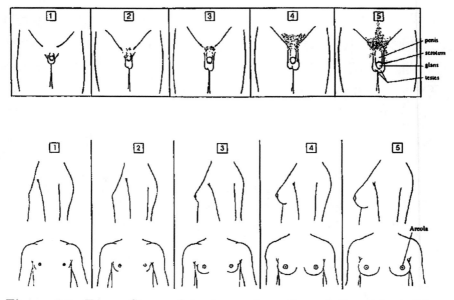

**Figure 3.1:** Tanner Stages of development one through five. Adapted from [127].

would be mostly grown, provided that the 11-year-old is Tanner Stage 2 and the 15-year-old is Tanner Stage 4 or 5 and has had her periods for at least two years [60, p. 56].

The way boys grow is slightly less straightforward to grasp, because they do not have a biological marker like menstruation to indicate where they are along their developmental path, and their pubertal changes start, on average, two years later than girls'. If you are used to Tanner (SMR) staging all patients as a matter of course and are able to explain it to parents, something most pediatricians should be able to do, you will not have to worry about averages, because you will know where a child is in his or her growth trajectory. Remember these SMR ratings or Tanner Stages, though, because they will figure prominently into how we figure "ideal body weight" in the chapter on outpatient care.

If a patient acquires anorexia nervosa during the growth phase (up to about 18 years for boys and 14 years for girls), linear growth can be stunted. Whether or not catch-up growth will ever entirely make up the deficit is not known. Brain growth, too, is affected by inadequate nutrition, and some brain-imaging studies have suggested that the deficit may never be entirely recovered [30] [65].

A word about social growth is in order here. All parents want their children to lead happy, fulfilled lives as adults. Essential to this goal are good relationships, commonly eventual marriage, and perhaps parenthood. Anorexia nervosa is a profoundly socially stunting disorder. Social withdrawal may be the first thing some parents notice. Eventually a child's preoccupation with weight, calories, food, and so on becomes so consuming they cease doing the social things they once did. If this is allowed to go on for years, social stunting is the rule.

## 3.2   Ascertaining the seriousness of weight loss

How much weight loss is serious? Isn't some weight loss a good thing? How can a parent convince their spouse or child or their insurance company to take their child's weight loss seriously? For that matter, how can they convince their pediatrician? These questions come up again and again. Pediatricians take note.

At the Kartini Clinic we have never heard a pediatrician criticized for overreacting to a child's weight loss, but we have had many, many complaints about doctors refusing to listen to parents' concerns about their child's weight loss. Sometimes a pediatrician will have conscientiously and accurately recorded the weight loss and subsequent flattening of the height curve, without seeming to have drawn any conclusions from it. Because the medical consequences of weight loss can be severe and sometimes even irreversible, this is a tenuous position for a pediatric provider to be in. In general, if a doctor or nurse practitioner suspects anorexia nervosa, or another eating disorder, they should refer the child to an experienced eating-disorder team, particularly if hospitalization may be needed. For this reason, an understanding of the standardized admission criteria published by the American Academy of Pediatrics is essential. Parents should be familiar with them and they should see to it that their child's therapists, nutritionists or doctors are too. Please review the American Academy of Pediatrics guidelines for admission to the hospital for children with eating disorders presented and discussed in the chapter on inpatient hospitalization, if you care for children and teens.

## 3.3   Common clinical presentations

### Syncope and pre-syncope (fainting)

Next to weight loss, syncopal episodes are the number one way for an eating-disordered child to present to the pediatrician's or family physician's office. If you are faced with a girl *or a boy* who has had a fainting episode and who has few or no other physical findings, please think of taking a food history before you order a cardiac consult. Then look at the patient's heart rate. If it is below 50, even in an athletic child, check their weight. If they have lost weight, strongly consider an urgent eating-disorder evaluation. An experienced eating-disorder physician is able to distinguish anorexia nervosa from other medical conditions and will be the first one to refer the patient to other specialties if the patient does not have an eating disorder.

# Food hoarding and bags of vomitus

As odd as it sounds, finding bags of vomitus under the bed or in the closet is not uncommon in eating-disordered patients. Sometimes the bags do not contain vomitus, but rather food that has been chewed and spit out. It is effectively the same thing. The pediatrician should quietly discuss such a finding with the child and the parent, minimizing the bizarre nature of this behavior in front of the child, and then refer them to an eating-disorder clinic. There are essentially no "normal" explanations for a child storing bags of vomitus in her/his room.

Occasionally what is found are bags or stashes of uneaten food or treats. This food hoarding can be a sign of binge eating or of enforced dieting (small children who are forced to diet or to restrict their sweets commonly hide food). Have the parents check the toilet and the shower for any signs of acid stomach contents. Have the parent check the room for diet pills or laxatives. If you think that the hoarding is being done because of overly strict enforcement of food rules at home, try to reason with the parent, as this is almost certain to be counterproductive and lead to secretive behaviors around food. You may need the help of a therapist or an eating-disorder physician to support you in helping the parents sort this one out.

# A sudden change in food habits

Vegetarians are sometimes offended by the suggestion that a choice to give up meat is a frequent precursor to anorexia nervosa, but this has been our consistent experience. Children report that they quit eating meat for the love of animals, something that it is difficult to argue with, but in fact this decision occurs almost always either simultaneous to or around the time of the onset of their eating problems. We have interviewed many patients in good remission about this decision (which we do not honor unless the vegetarianism clearly preceded the eating disorder or the family are lifelong vegetarians), and they have confirmed our suspicion that their decision not to eat meat had been all about reducing fat. If patients are allowed to be vegans, their re-feeding is almost impossible to manage. Many will also claim "lactose intolerance," again something they later tell us was about the anxiety they experienced eating or drinking dairy products (which contain fats). Some assuage their anxiety by making certain that all of their dairy products are fat-free, but for some that is not radical enough. We try not to argue about the lactose intolerance, but merely matter-of-factly provide them with Lactaid. They usually do not want to go to the trouble of using the Lactaid in the long run and become miraculously cured of their lactose intolerance. True lactose intolerance exists, of course, but there should be a history of it preceding the onset of the eating disorder. Beware of diagnosing lactose intolerance because it "runs in the family," as eating disorders also "run in the family," and it is not unusual to have another family member (often a parent) engaging in restricting behavior. If it becomes imperative to find out, refer the patient for lactose testing.

A common story for parents to relate to their pediatrician is that their child first decided to cut out all fast food for the sake of health—laudable enough. Then they decided to become a vegetarian, and then they cut back on their portions, claiming to have stomach aches, to be too full, or to have already eaten elsewhere. When confronted, the child may insist that they would eat if their parents would just make the food they like, but when the parents do, the child either doesn't eat it, eats only a small part of it, or comes up with more excuses. Soon school lunches are discovered petrifying in a locker, or the child becomes thinner and thinner while the family dog becomes fatter and fatter!

## A dramatic increase in exercise

If giving up fast food is something that seems praiseworthy to many observers, imagine how they feel about a child's sudden—even extreme—interest in exercise. Former couch potatoes begin to go to the gym: Everyone is pleased! Children who are already athletic begin to work out rigorously outside of their team training. They may aspire to train for the Olympics and draw their proud parents into this plan. Even if I wanted to speak out against too much exercise (to the detriment of a person's social, emotional, intellectual, and spiritual development), it is quite simply true that exercise is the sacred cow of current American life, and you cannot imply that there could be too much of this good thing as long as we all "know" that American children are fatter than ever before. Parents and (especially) physicians are sometimes unable to gain a balanced perspective about exercise and weight loss, because quite often they, too, wish they had the "self-control" to do as the eating-disordered child is doing. To approach this sensibly, parent and physician need to be sure that if the exercise has taken a dramatic upturn, then so must the caloric intake, including the intake of heart-healthy fats.

## Vocal concern about weight, fat, and size

Very young children with anorexia nervosa are often the most honest and open about what is going on with them. If they feel they are fat, they will say so openly, again and again. Older children, having read about eating disorders in the press, may be too sophisticated to admit, "I think I am fat" or "I don't deserve to eat," but they often write this in their journals and talk about it to their friends. Anorexia nervosa being a brain disorder, however, they will almost certainly not be able to stop themselves from talking at some point about their own and other people's size. Sometimes this concern is disguised by an obsession with being "toned," "having a six-pack," or "being in shape." One day a parent may wake up and realize that size and food have become the topic of conversation almost all the time.

## Social withdrawal

Anorexia nervosa is a profoundly isolating disease. Even though patients who were fat before the onset of their illness report an initial improvement in their social lives as people respond to their slim selves more positively, they eventually become so obsessed with avoiding food, exercising, or purging (if they do that) that they spend even less time with their friends. They may spend a lot of time alone in their rooms, or prefer to walk to and from school even in terrible weather rather than join their friends. They may avoid social situations where food will be served and their nonparticipation commented on. They may simply become too tired to enjoy the full social life they once did.

## Avoiding family meals

Most parents begin to get worried when they see their child pushing food around on their plate and eating only a small amount of what they were served, and that's *if* the family eats meals together at all. A child may claim to have too much homework and to want to eat in his or her room. In my experience, almost all patients who have severe anorexia nervosa eventually try to avoid eating around others. An exception to this may be the child who is unafraid to eat with the family because they are assured they can rid themselves of any calories ingested by purging afterward. Young patients tell me it was initially to avoid comments from their parents that they wanted to eat alone, but that later they came to want to savor in private the small amount of food they allowed themselves. Some patients comment that they became fearful that others would think they ate too much; other patients report having become intensely disturbed by people chewing.

## Becoming a family chef

When humans are starved, their brains become focused on food. This makes perfect sense, since in any animal, during a time of famine, the ones most focused on food-seeking are most likely to survive. Consequently children with eating disorders become very food-focused. Contrary to what many people think (and what many patients initially try to say), anorexia nervosa is not about a lack of appetite. People with anorexia nervosa are hungry all the time, they think about food, and they may dream about food. Many become gourmet cooks, cooking and baking for friends and family, though not eating what they cook themselves. They may begin watching cooking shows on TV, reading cookbooks, collecting recipes, and cutting out food coupons. Boys may do this as well as girls, something even more striking.

One of our twelve-year-old male patients told us he went through a stage of creating elaborate and calorie-rich milkshakes for his younger brother, who was then forced to drink them while the older boy watched. As a 17-year-old girl put it, "I feel superior to other people because I eat less than they do."

## Mood instability

Imagine what would happen if you took a roomful of healthy men, gathered together to watch a football game, and deprived them of food for a day. It would not take long them to become very cranky. We are all like that. Mood instability often improves markedly with re-feeding in the hospital. The most common comment we hear from parents after a week of adequate caloric intake in the hospital is: "I have my child back."

## Psychogenic drinking

It is very common for our patients to present in what we refer to as a "water-loaded" state. We confirm this state routinely by checking the specific gravity (concentration) of their urine. 1.010 is suspicious, especially early in the morning, and 1.005 or less is almost confirmatory. Psychogenic drinking in its extreme form can cause hyponatremia and even seizures. One of our patients urinated off ten pounds of fluid a few hours after admission to the hospital. She had water loaded to increase her weight on our scales by going into bathroom in our office, putting her mouth under the tap, and turning it on. She hoped we would think she was washing her hands. We are rarely fooled by such behavior, but imagine how easy it would be to be fooled in a general pediatric office where people do not suspect it. Someone weighing such a patient might believe she had gained weight—which was the idea, of course.

There may be other reasons for this polydipsia (increased drinking) as well. Most of the so-called health magazines today have completely lost the idea of drinking to thirst, something our organism is exquisitely programmed to do; instead they suggest that the more you drink, the "cleaner" your insides and your kidneys are. Drinking water is promoted for weight loss. All over this country people are carrying plastic water bottles with them as if this were the Sahara. And, of course, drinking water or diet, calorie-free beverages is a way of suppressing appetite. For those patients whose heart rate is very low, drinks containing caffeine, like many of the "energy drinks" and diet sodas, jolt their hearts into a higher rate and they feel better, without knowing why. This is like flogging an ailing horse, of course, but it sustains them for a while.

There may be two other reasons for increased drinking: The thirst-control centers in and near the hypothalamus may be near parts of the brain affected by anorexia nervosa, reflecting possible hypothalamic dysfunction of water regulation [84]; and many patients have been put on an SSRI (selective serotonin reuptake inhibitor) medication such as Prozac or Paxil, which can itself cause increased thirst.

## 3.4 Common physical manifestations

### Bradycardia (low heart rate)

The issue of bradycardia in the setting of an eating disorder is relatively straightforward, although it sometimes gets mired in irrational controversy. The Academy of Pediatrics [1] recommends hospitalization for patients whose heart rate is less than 45 BPM (beats per minute) at night or 50 BPM during the day. Except when we have reason to believe that we have not gotten a true daytime (office hours) resting heart rate, either because of *anxiety, caffeine,* or *diet pills*, we adhere to these guidelines. In the case of an anxious child who just drank a latte or a diet Mountain Dew with a heart rate of 50—55 BPM along with other conditions of concern such as weight loss and behaviors consistent with anorexia nervosa, we put them in the hospital for observation overnight, as we are pretty sure the nighttime heart rate will be substantially lower once the stimulants wash out.

So where's the controversy? Every eating-disorder physician has had the experience of putting such a child in the hospital only to have someone tell the family, "Oh, that heart rate of 40 is not a problem—your child is an athlete. Why, Lance Armstrong's resting heart rate is in the 30s." Worried parents may then begin to doubt our decision to hospitalize. Let's be clear: Pediatric patients, even the very athletic ones, are not adult athletes. It is not that we think a child with a heart rate in the 30s or 40s will die overnight (though this has been reported [85] [46]) but that *this clear parameter allows us to get immediate inpatient help for a patient we are sure needs stabilization for their eating disorder.* Furthermore, if these extremely low heart rates were somehow normal for this athletic child, they would not correct with re-feeding, which they *always* do. We have never yet had a patient whose heart rate did not get above 50 BPM once they were stabilized medically. We make no assertion about what a heart rate of 50 BPM may mean in a healthy, non-dieting adult.

If you can do only one thing in your office to evaluate the need for referral in a child you are worried about, make that one thing taking a resting heart rate. So simple. Have the child lie down, put a blanket over them, and wait five or ten minutes. Do not weigh them first (which may trigger anxiety) or discuss weight, if it can be helped.

# Hypothermia $(T < 96°F)$

This least dramatic of all vital signs may one day turn out to be the most interesting. Our patients are nearly uniformly hypothermic. As outpatients they report being cold. Once re-feeding is started and their metabolism increases, they may complain about being hot, even sweating profusely, but their core temperature often remains cold. It makes intuitive sense that an emaciated patient with little subcutaneous fat to insulate them would be hypothermic, but why do they often remain so when weight restored? Perhaps the hypothalamic control of temperature is telling us something about which parts of the brain are affected or co-affected.

## Orthostasis (cardiovascular instability)

The American Academy of Pediatrics considers a pulse differential of 20 BPM or greater from lying to standing to be "orthostatic." When testing for this "orthostasis," have the patient lie down for five minutes and then stand for two and a half minutes to avoid the first flash of "standing up too fast." If the differential is 20—34 BPM and they are otherwise medically stable, we may choose to give a can of Ensure © or Boost © and watch closely over the next few days. If there is a 35 BPM differential or more, we hospitalize them. Again, we are not frightened by this number, but rather regard it as a *marker for degree of eating-disorder destabilization*. We certainly don't want anyone to faint and knock out their adult teeth. If the patient is this orthostatic, they need to be in the hospital for the induction of re-feeding (something that we feel cannot be done at home either safely or efficiently) and/or for enforced abstinence from any purging.

## Amenorrhea (lack of menstruation)

Amenorrhea, although it can and eventually will have a deleterious effect on the bones, should not be used as a criterion for establishing the diagnosis of anorexia nervosa for several reasons: The patient may be male, the patient may be prepubertal, if the patient is a female she may never yet have achieved regularity to her periods, she may be on birth control pills, she may be lying about having a period because she knows what it means for establishing weight goals, and, finally, amenorrhea has other causes. Furthermore, parents and patients often have family beliefs or common experience that cloud the discussion of a girl's period, such as "Mom didn't get her period until she was 17" (makes us wonder about Mom's eating-disorder history as a young girl), or "I never had regular periods anyway" (makes us wonder how long her eating disorder has actually been going on).

A plea to all doctors: In the face of a history consistent with an eating disorder, resist the temptation to send your patient to the gynecologist for a workup. This will often result in your patient being given oral contraceptives, which will only *apparently* help, and you will lose a valuable marker of biologic normalcy. Despite a long history of benefit to bone health in menopausal women, administration of hormones, or oral contraceptives, does *not* improve bone density in women with anorexia nervosa and should not be done [83] [36]. If the patient is very emaciated and reports regular periods, "trust but verify" by asking her mother whether she has ever seen proof of this assertion (not just disappearing tampons) or by getting an estradiol level, LH and FSH (female

hormone levels). If the estradiol is less than 30 pg/ml and the FSH
and LH are very low, be deeply skeptical of a history of normal
menses [37].

## Carotenemia (orange skin color)

Carotenemia, like the carotenemia of infancy, is a harmless, in-
cidental finding often seen in our patients, especially those who
consume large amounts of carrots, yams, pumpkins or carrot juice.
I mention it because you may see it.

## Russell's sign

Russell's Sign is a physical finding to be noted in the chart, but not
something with which a doctor would want to confront, embarrass,
or scold the patient. Russell's sign consists of skin changes, often
small scars or calluses, over the knuckle of the index and middle
finger on the dominant hand, and comes from repeatedly using
the hand to induce vomiting. It is a piece of the puzzle only and
can be absent even with significant vomiting.

## Tooth erosion

If a doctor is good at examining the teeth (I am not), he/she may
see tooth erosion where the patient has a history of ridding herself
of food by vomiting. If there is any doubt, as part of the patient's
general care, the doctor should refer her/him to a dentist and
alert the dentist (with the family's permission) to the suspicion
of purging. If the child freely admits to vomiting, a dental exam
might still be in order for further dental care suggestions.

## Swollen glands

All textbooks mention swollen glands, and when present they are easy to see, but what I see more often than discrete swollen parotid glands is more a diffuse fullness to the jaw area. This can become permanent with fibrotic changes from years of purging.

# 3.5   Common laboratory findings

In evaluating for an eating disorder, lab tests are the least significant thing a doctor can do in the office. *Vitals, exam,* and *history* are much more important. In fact, physicians have often been falsely consoled by "normal labs." In restricting anorexia lab tests may be normal even in the face of a patient so ill they require admission to an intensive care unit. Despite what one might think, our patients rarely have anemia or low blood proteins. In more severe cases they may have neutropenia (a low white blood cell count) or have slightly elevated liver enzymes. Electrolytes will usually be normal unless the patient is purging a lot. To evaluate for the possibility of purging, look for elevated $CO_2$ (even if still technically in the high normal range) and depressed chloride (even if still technically in the low normal range). Check phosphorus levels, if you are going to do labs. More about the details of these numbers is reviewed in the section on inpatient hospitalization.

## The REDS-Child (rating of eating disorder severity) semi-structured interview

Eating-disorder physicians all use some form of structured, semi-structured, or self-report interview to help make a diagnosis and to distinguish between anorexia and other eating disorders. The one we use and have liked for years (the REDS) was developed for adults by Dr. Eliot Goldner of Vancouver, British Columbia, and modified by me for use with children (REDS-C). (See Appendix A.) It is a semi-structured interview that requires the doctor to ask questions and grade the answers. It includes a score for severity of symptoms as well as a confidence in the veracity of each response. A high score indicates severe symptomatology, and a high confidence score indicates the interviewer's belief that the answers given were truthful. Both scores can be reported as a composite, or each answer can be analyzed on its own merits. The parameters being scored are: Degree of caloric restriction, variety of foods eaten, discomfort eating around others, presence/absence of bingeing, frequency of bingeing, presence/absence of purging (vomiting, laxatives, etc.), frequency of purging, degree of compensatory exercise, BMI (as an indication of degree of cachexia), cognitive drive for thinness, denial of seriousness of weight loss/low body weight, social effect of eating behaviors, body image distortion, and medical effect of the eating behaviors. The confidence scoring allows us to look back and examine each question individually in light of how reliable the interviewer felt the answer to be.

Each eating-disorder treatment center has its favorite instrument to use to assess severity of illness or establish diagnosis. Few are useful for the general practitioner. Our practitioners like the REDS-C because self-report questionnaires are felt to be impersonal and unreliable, especially with very young children, and because the REDS-C includes a medical component. The semi-structured nature of the REDS-C is also a way of being certain that a complete history is taken, and its more open structure gives latitude to ask many more detailed, open-ended questions than a self-report instrument typically covers. The REDS-C is, of course, time-consuming and is done as part of the approximately two-hour interview of child and family that is routine in our specialty clinic.

A copy of the REDS-C is included in the back of this book for the reader's interest.

## 3.6   Other medical disorders presenting as weight loss

**Cognitive deficits:** One small group of patients who present with weight loss is hardly ever discussed. About half a dozen times in my career as an eating-disorder doctor I have been asked to evaluate a patient with significant weight loss who struck me as clearly not fulfilling any of the criteria for an eating disorder. Furthermore, once I interviewed the patient I began to wonder about their intellectual functioning. Testing in these cases revealed IQs in the borderline mentally retarded range around 60-70. These children were socially adept enough to mask their impaired intellectual capabilities. They were quite simply in need of an adult in their life taking responsibility for regularly doing the shopping and cooking meals, something that has become rarer and rarer in our rushed society. In the past, when most mothers were home and fixing all meals, such children would not have presented with weight loss. These patients were able to be quickly returned to their premorbid weight once the correct diagnosis was made and their parents understood what the problem was. No eating disorder was present.

**Brain tumors:** Brain tumors may also present with weight loss, although in my experience such patients rarely fulfill the psychological criteria for anorexia nervosa and any vomiting is more eruptive and less controlled. A person with bulimia or purging anorexia will almost never vomit in bed or all over themselves. Suffice it to say, a careful neurological exam is an essential part of every eating-disorder workup, paying special attention to the cranial nerves. The tumors I have seen were all brain stem tumors, in both males and females, except for one neurofibroma in a patient with neurofibromatosis (von Recklinghausen disease), but the literature reports many other types [73] [71] [43] [19]. If eating-disorder evaluation by an eating-disorder specialist must be delayed, an MRI (not CT) is indicated whenever there is any doubt. MRI will more clearly delineate the brain stem.

**Addison's disease:** We have had one adolescent patient who presented with vomiting, weight loss, and syncope who clearly was not eating disordered once her REDS-C score had been rated by us. A careful review of her history led me to suspect Addison's Disease (primary adrenal failure). Her parents were informed, and a pediatric endocrinologist confirmed that this was the case. Addison's Disease is quite rare, but should always be in the back of the doctor's mind as the doctor works through the differential diagnosis of a patient with weight loss and vomiting.

**Munchhausen by proxy:** This is a rare condition. I have had two cases to date, both in adopted children whose mothers were the perpetrators. For "reasons" one can only surmise, these mothers were vested in convincing the treating team that the child had anorexia nervosa and "refused to eat." The first patient was a very young girl adopted from India. Eventually we became suspicious when the child exhibited no anxiety whatsoever about what we fed her in the clinic. Whenever she was sent home, her mother returned with tales of how she neither ate nor drank despite all of Mom's (carefully described) interventions. The child was very thin, but she exhibited little weight loss and ate voraciously when food was offered. She was unable (unwilling) to tell us what was going on at home, and only the intervention of a multidisciplinary team was finally able to uncover the truth. When confronted, the mother left the state. The other case was in an older adolescent whose adoptive mother insisted that her child was fat or going to become so from "compulsive over-eating." When we could not be convinced that her child was bingeing, she began to restrict her child's access to all food even to the extent of refusing to let her leave the home for fear she would "eat at other people's homes." Fortunately this child was old enough to tell us exactly what was happening and frightened enough by her adoptive mother's mental illness that she requested foster placement.

## 3.7   A word about parents

Even though the literature on eating disorders is replete with stories of "parents in denial," it has been our experience that parents generally do a better job than we doctors at recognizing that "something is wrong" with their child. Perhaps we should not be surprised. Parents are the experts on their own children and, with very few exceptions, should be treated as such. Anorexia nervosa is a life- and health-threatening condition, and parents who have grounds to feel something is not right should not be made to feel invasive if they look through their children's rooms or bathrooms for evidence of vomiting, food hoarding, diet pills, syrup of ipecac (which "novices" use to induce vomiting), or laxatives. I do advise parents to have a word with themselves before any such search, however, and if they find love letters from unsuitable admirers, condoms, homework assignments with bad grades, and so forth, not to use this search as a springboard to confront their child with everything they disapprove of. Stick to the life-threatening stuff. Deal with the rest later.

Physicians, if a parent insists that their child's weight loss is a problem, please do not brush them off. Take a history. Be sure of your diagnosis. If parents insist that they are concerned that their normally social child is now only exercising and doing homework, think back to the initial presentation of anorexia nervosa described by Richard Morton reported in Chapter 1. A young doctor who ignores the concerns of mothers or grandmothers is foolish; an older doctor who does so is just a plain fool.

## Clinical pearls

- Weight loss in childhood is not normal, until proven otherwise.

- Failure to gain weight is "weight loss" in a growing child.

- Fat children get anorexia, too! It is not a good trade-off.

- Common presentations are fainting, sudden change in food habits, food hoarding, bags of vomitus, vocal concern about fat and size, dramatic increase in exercise, social withdrawal though grades are often intact, cooking enthusiastically for others but not eating any themselves, avoiding family meals, mood instability, psychogenic drinking, and weight loss.

- DO NOT wait more than a week to see a child back in your office about whom you are concerned.

# 4 Eating disorders of childhood

From the point of view of a desperate or scared parent or concerned grandparent, the kind who calls the Kartini Clinic every day for advice, exactly which eating disorder their own child has matters less than how it is going to be treated. But it does matter. As in all other branches of medicine, we are determined to diagnose a condition as accurately as we can because prognosis (outcome) may be affected. As an example, it is important to know whether a patient has primary cancer of the bone or cancer which has metastasized (spread) to the bone from a different cancer elsewhere, because prognosis and treatment will vary.

Does my child have bulimia nervosa or anorexia nervosa with vomiting? How does it matter?

Having said that, needless hair-splitting such as occurs during discussions of DSM (Diagnostic and Statistical Manual of Mental Disorders) categories between professionals may not reflect actual clinically relevant groups of patients. Some day it may serve us well to divide what is currently called bulimia, anorexia, and EDNOS (eating disorder not otherwise specified) into "restricting eating disorder" or "purging eating disorder." This would effectively help drain the swamp of EDNOS and facilitate research.

Classification systems of mental illnesses should actually be called *recognizable patterns of human brain dysfunction*, as that is what they are. Recognizable patterns. For most mental illnesses, there is no litmus test, no lab study or X-ray that will make the diagnosis. Not yet, anyway. That is why careful observation, awareness of what the patterns look like in other children, and listening to parents as the best historians we have, is so critical. There is a lot of discussion and argumentation going on right now about the fine details of DSM classification in the world of eating disorders. For the sake of clarity and clinical usefulness, I will cover the five most common in a pediatric eating disorder clinic: Anorexia nervosa (including those who binge and/or purge and may be referred to as "anorexia AND bulimia" by others), bulimia nervosa, selective eating, food phobia/functional dysphagia, and imitative forms ("dieting gone awry"). My view of these categories will, of course, be represented here. Some practitioners will have other names for the same or similar things. Right now we care about getting a sensible understanding of which eating disorder a child has, debunking any blaming (including self-blaming), and deciding what needs to be done next to keep the child safe, to give them their life back and the parents their child back.

A general pediatrician, pediatric nurse practitioner, or family physician can make the diagnosis of an eating disorder in their office, bearing in mind the previous chapter's discussion of "presentation" and using a few simple observations and tests.

In a specialized pediatric eating disorder clinic such as the Kartini Clinic, the overwhelming majority of patients under 18 years of age will l have anorexia nervosa or a subclinical variant that doesn't quite meet all DSM IV (Fourth edition) criteria. These variants are formally known as "Eating Disorder Not Otherwise Specified" (EDNOS). Oh, you can't imagine how much arguing among professionals goes on over this category (EDNOS)! For our purposes, however, let us agree to call anorexia nervosa all cases of self-induced food restriction that result in weight loss or failure to gain weight, with or without body dysmorphism (known to be absent in some younger children and/or males). EDNOS, in my opinion, is best reserved for those cases that do not fit either the anorexia profile nor the bulimia profile. Rather, conditions which cannot be categorized at all and which an experienced clinician cannot see as progressing to either.

Sound confusing? It is. Perhaps the most useful exercise would be to dispense with this category altogether. Clinically, only *pattern recognition* matters, because the pattern will likely point us in the direction of clinical course and from there to outcome.

In an inpatient setting, the percentage of children with anorexia nervosa or EDNOS (as others prefer to call cases not meeting strict DSM-IV criteria) is well above 90%. Yet bulimia nervosa (9.9 cases per year per 100,000 population) is more common in the general population than anorexia nervosa (6.3 per year per 100,000 people) [47], so why don't we see it very often at the Kartini Clinic?

Bulimia nervosa (BN) is probably a less medically compromising condition than restricting anorexia nervosa or purging anorexia nervosa. BN often goes either undisclosed and undiagnosed or is treated successfully in a psychological practice with the support of an SSRI and hence never makes it to specialty medical attention. It is less common in young children (explaining why we see less of it). If a doctors looks for it in his or her general practice, or makes him or herself open to the discussion of body image issues, he or she will definitely see it.

Distinguishing between bulimia nervosa and purging or binge/purging anorexia nervosa can be challenging. It is important, though, because in our clinical experience the prognosis appears to be different, with what is called BN having a more benign course [86]. As a rule of thumb, patients with BN are of normal or higher-than-normal body weight and will not have experienced the prolonged periods of very low body weight that patients with purging anorexia experience. The late Peter Beumont of the University of Sydney felt this was an important clinical distinction to make (personal communication) and I agree. People with purging anorexia nervosa may have periods of time where they primarily restrict followed by periods of time where their pattern shifts to primarily bingeing and purging. I do not think this means their diagnosis has changed; their illness is merely cycling in a predictable way. Again: These are recognizable patterns.

The pediatric practitioner is almost certain to run into a case of food phobia (functional dysphagia) at least once. For a discussion of this entity, please see below.

Selective eating (also described below) is very common in a general pediatric practice, but is usually handled by generalists so well that we see only the most refractory cases. This is as it should be. I hope the information below will serve as a guide to parents searching for a greater understanding of the variants of disordered eating that can occur in childhood. The rest of the book will overwhelmingly focus on anorexia nervosa, both restricting and binge/purging variants, as these are the conditions associated with the greatest burden of medical complications and—yes—even death.

## 4.1   Anorexia nervosa

I will not spend much time more debating the criteria for anorexia nervosa put forth by the DSM IV except to mention that 1) by the time a committee of clinicians and scholars have met, dissected, and voted on criteria for a brain disorder (mental illness) and the book has been published, it is already out of date, and 2) to date, iterations of the DSM have addressed mostly adults, and modifications for children are weak at best. As Dasha Nicholls and Bryan Lask, then of Great Ormond Street hospital for Children in London, so aptly put it, "Children into DSM don't go!" [86]

However, there are basically four criteria which must be met to make the diagnosis of anorexia nervosa, according to the DSM, and all of them are flawed as criteria for children in a clinical setting. I review them here so that you may defend yourselves against practitioners or insurers who tell you your child or your patient "doesn't have an eating disorder" based on "not meeting DSM criteria."

**1. Weight loss or failure to gain weight such that the patient's weight is less than 85% of expected body weight.**

Like any disease or illness, anorexia nervosa must start somewhere. When a 10-year-old child has lost 15% of his or her body weight, he or she will be very sick indeed. There is no reason to wait until a child has met this criterion, and there is every reason not to wait. Just remember: *Weight loss in childhood is not normal and must be considered a problem until proven otherwise, irrespective of the premorbid weight.* In other words, if a fat child presents to you behaviors you would call eating disordered in a slender child, you have a problem *even if they are still fat.* I cannot tell you how often we are presented with children who have lost catastrophic amounts of weight, as much as 40% of their body weight, and yet because they are "not thin" are not referred for help. An example of this was a fourteen year old girl who was 5 feet 3 inches tall and weighed 220 pounds before she became anorexic. Once her severe weight loss was noticed and referred she weighed 150 pounds (32% of her body weight been lost). She was weak, fainting, bradycardic (low heart rate) and cold. But her doctor thought she was "fine," in fact, "better off."

This discussion is not intended to minimize the consequences of obesity in children, merely a plea to think things through: If a child had a malignant tumor that caused this degree of weight loss, few people would argue that such a child was "better off" because they were now thinner. Be careful what you say!

At the Kartini Clinic, we use our own first criterion to help define anorexia nervosa of childhood: "Unexplained weight loss or failure to gain weight in a child whose age and Tanner Stage (SMR) would lead you to expect continued growth" or "persistent weight loss in a child whose growth has ceased."

**2. Intense fear of fat despite low weight (may be absent).**

**3. Disturbance in the way in which body weight or shape is experienced *or* the patient shows undue influence of weight on their self-evaluation *or* reveals denial of the seriousness of their low body weight or weight loss.**

These are generally good criteria and probably often pertain even when the patient denies them, but they are also fraught with difficulty. Young children, depending on their age and stage of development, vary greatly in their ability to think abstractly and to put their thoughts—concrete or abstract—into words. Some very young patients will present right away with the delusional belief that they are fat, despite all evidence to the contrary, or they may express a paranoid fear of being made fat by their caretakers. I call this "the adult form of the disease," and some young children have it. But others either do not experience a frank fear of fat or are unable to conceptualize it as such. They may merely appear to be sad. In their innocence of calories and fat grams, very young children may actually eat things older people with anorexia would never touch (i.e. fat-containing foods). It is their extreme resistance to food in general that gives them away. They may hide food or simply sit and cry (they rarely purge). Their distress is difficult to elicit in a diagnostic interview and may be better approached through art therapy or what we call "longitudinal experience" with the child: i.e. spending more time observing. The disease, if present, will eventually rear its ugly head.

Assessing the value of the "influence of weight or shape on (a child's) self-evaluation" may also be distorted by the child's family experience. Many, many adults are dieting, and many more are either going to the gym "to get fit" or talking about doing it. A young child could easily be forgiven if they got the idea from adults that they "are what they look like." We spend little time convincing children that character and intellect are as important to who they are as what they look like. If you take a rigorous look at the effect of body weight and shape on the self-evaluation of (non-eating-disordered) women today, I think you would be hard pressed to find this a consistently meaningful sorting point [76] [119].

**4. Amenorrhea.**

Obviously amenorrhea pertains only to those old enough to have regular periods and to females. This is an important clinical observation, but, in my opinion, a worthless criterion, a bit like making amenorrhea a criterion for diagnosing pregnancy: The literature is replete with stories of women who menstruate throughout the first months of pregnancy, and there are eating disordered patients whose weight is critically low but who continue to menstruate. Such patients, despite the absence of amenorrhea, have a similar course of illness.

# AN subtypes

There are two important subtypes of AN : The restricting subtype and the purging or binge-purging subtype.

Restricting anorexia nervosa is the most common form in early childhood—so much so that when we first developed our Day Treatment Unit (DTU) for children with eating disorders, we developed it for "restrictors" only. We felt that homogeneity of the milieu was an important goal (described at length in Chapter 12), and only a small number of patients did not fit this category (restrictors). Once we began seeing older adolescents, and especially once we included those between the ages of 18 and 22 years, though, those numbers changed dramatically. To serve all the children we found it necessary to create another DTU program to attend to the needs of those who suffered from the bingeing and purging subtype of anorexia. Eventually, we combined the DTU's, but still work hard to keep the diagnostic groups separate for most interventions.

Therapists who work with eating-disordered patients will tell you that the two populations ("restrictors" and "purgers," here so noted for the sake of clarity, though we never refer to patients themselves like this) differ dramatically in presentation and in temperament. Children who restrict their intake but do not binge or purge seem to be characterized by *behavioral over-control*: For the most part they are very compliant, they are pleasers, they do well with adults, they are focused on school achievement, and they tend to be high achievers, strivers, and socially conformist. They typically do not take drugs, do not engage in risky sexual behaviors, and do not cut on themselves. In short, they are not *impulsive*. Physicians often like to work with these kids because they tend to "do what they're told." Therapists, however, often find them more of a challenge because they are more constricted in their range of affect and are therefore harder to draw out.

The parents of such children (who restrict only) have usually been challenged very little by their children; these are the "perfect children" who "never caused trouble." One effect of this temperament type on treatment can be parental reluctance to believe that their heretofore perfect child might exercise secretly or throw away food and lie about it. Additionally, their parents may have had little experience setting limits with such "easy" children, making the parental control over meals very challenging for them.

We once worked with a father, a prominent attorney, whose daughter had restricting anorexia. She had a hard time gaining the required weight as an outpatient because she hid food and threw away her lunches. Of course she told her Dad she did not. In other words, she lied. The family therapist tried to frame this obvious (to us) lying as something "anorexia was doing," not the child, but the father became very angry. He began yelling at the therapist and accused the program of "not trusting his child whom he knew to have been honest all her life." He stalked out, taking his daughter with him, only to return a week later and apologize when her lunches had been found uneaten at her school. We tried to help him understand that it was necessary to differentiate between attacking the behavior and attacking the child. But he had a hard time with this as his child "had never lied before."

The behaviors associated with purging or binge-purging anorexia are often quite different. The parents of the children with this variant of AN may not have the same difficulty as the father just described because their children have challenged them more. These patients seem to have a different brain chemistry, one often characterized by *impulsivity*. We frequently see self-destructive behaviors such as cutting, experimenting with or even frankly abusing alcohol or drugs, and of course, vomiting. Physicians may have a harder time managing these patients who challenge their authority more, but therapists enjoy working with these kids because they are frequently more forthcoming, "in your face," and individualistic. Like their "restrictor" counterparts, they are often perfectionistic and excellent students—but not always.

Parents read about eating disorders in books and on the Web. Increasingly they write their own blogs and participate in online forums. It is a common misunderstanding to feel that being a "restrictor" is somehow "better" than being a "purger." If their child has not purged for a long time, parents may resist having their child's eating disorder categorized as "purging variant anorexia nervosa" and demand that we re-categorize their child as having "restricting variant" and place them in the "restrictor group" in the Day Treatment Unit. We try to explain that children who have ever purged, whether regularly or not, need to feel free to discuss this behavior without feeling judged. In fact, contrary to popular misunderstanding, we separate the two groups by diagnosis not to protect the restrictors from contagion by those who purge, but rather to protect those who purge from the harsh judgment of those who do not. And while there seems to be little doubt that the prognosis for severe, chronic purging anorexia can be one of the worst, we have seen several patients with this variant of the disorder do well when their parents are in good coalition with the treatment team while another patient with restricting anorexia nervosa whose family refuses to believe she is as "sick as the others" never quite gets into remission and hence does poorly [27].

There is a widespread belief that "restrictors" eventually turn into "purgers" or that many do. Does this happen? I do not see older adults and so cannot confirm this, but I do have my doubts. I wonder whether or not some people with a long history of restricting don't just later suffer from the bingeing known to follow prolonged starvation. And then, once finding themselves compelled (by the brain) to binge, may find vomiting the logical way to control their intake. These patients will remain "behaviorally over-controlled" as described above and not go on to engage in other impulsive behaviors. I wonder whether or not they would have experienced the bingeing had their weight restoration been more "structured" (see discussion of our meal plan).

Given that twin studies suggest that self-induced vomiting is highly heritable [117], it seems unlikely to me that the genetics of these differing disorders change, although there are certainly adult eating-disorder specialists who report this "switch."

## 4.2 Bulimia nervosa

At the Kartini Clinic we see patients with bulimia nervosa (BN), as mentioned above, though mostly in an outpatient or day treatment setting. Many people refer to everything that includes vomiting as "bulimia," but this is not accurate. Bulimia nervosa involves bingeing on large amounts of food and then getting rid of the food by vomiting, but it is not characterized by *prolonged* episodes of starvation such that weight is suppressed over months or years. People with bulimia nervosa are usually either normal weight or even heavier than normal. If a person has restricted and starved for any length of time and has consequently lost a significant amount of weight, they have, by definition, the purging or binge-purging variant of anorexia.

Bulimia is a miserable condition to have, but seems to respond well to psychotherapy (CBT), the support of an SSRI, and ordered eating [26] [91]. Bingeing and its consequence (purging) is kept alive by erratic eating habits that often include skipping breakfast and/or lunch followed by ravenous hunger in the late afternoon and evening. A study was done in Australia by Touyz, Beumont, *et al.* showing that group therapy could be effective treatment for BN as well [15]. It has been our experience that bulimia is rare in children under 13.

## 4.3 Selective eating

Selective eating is definitely something that a pediatric or family medicine provider will see in their practice. These are the children who eat only a very narrow range of foods, for example: peanut butter, pineapple, white bread with no crust, and a certain brand of noodles with spaghetti sauce. They are the despair of their grandparents; parents feel tremendous guilt about not being able to "talk their kids into eating better," or "punish them into it," depending on their school of thought. And these food preferences are bomb-proof. The children are rarely amenable to talking or cajoling, much less punishing. The more you push, the more they resist.

When confronted with such a child or their desperate parents, most pediatricians break out the growth chart, and this, I believe, is the correct response. If the child makes it as far as our eating-disorder clinic, this is exactly what we will do. Remember: *First, do no harm.* If you are a clinician asked to evaluate a child with selective eating, do a physical, listen respectfully to the mother or father, get a series of normal labs (if you must) to reassure the parents—but most of all listen, take a family history, and look at the growth chart. If the growth chart is normal and the child is not losing weight and growing in height, you are in safe waters.

Selective eating runs in families and is one of the few eating disorders that is more common in boys. My experience is that if you look around in the family, you will find an adult male who also has it. I say "has it" rather than "had it" because it seems to persist throughout life, although adults are more adept at hiding it or adjusting their lives to it. You may discover that Dad eats only steak, certain kinds of hamburger with no relish, potatoes, and broccoli with no dressing. His wife will have adjusted to this with a sigh, his doctors will never have taken a food history so they'll never know, and he will have figured out which restaurants he can visit. But a child is less able to design his environment and so gets "caught out." That's where the growth chart comes in: If growth is good, everything is good. Reassure the parents that they are doing a good job. Reassure the child that he or she is a great kid, name the disorder, find some humor in it, and identify his or her relative (if any) who also has it so that he or she does not feel like "a freak." Offer to explain selective eating to concerned grandparents who may be peppering the parents with behavioral advice. Usually this will be enough for everyone to feel reassured. Selective eating is not going to go away, so you might as well focus on what matters: The child's growth.

If the family simply cannot be reassured by this, we have them meet with our family therapist at regular intervals (weekly) and keep a food journal of what the child eats every day. Our doctors see the child every month or so to monitor weight and height changes. After several months of this, even the most worried parents can usually be reassured that they have done all they could to be sure they are not adversely affecting their child's growth.

Once I had a patient referred to me from the United Kingdom. He was a young man of 23 and had had selective eating all of his life. He wanted to go on a trip abroad, and truly wanted to be able to eat a wider variety of food with his friends. He really did. He came with his Dad, and I explained all of the above to them. They were relieved that this did not indicate some terrible hidden psychopathology in this seemingly well-adjusted, somewhat shy young man, and there was a positive family history for selective eating in an uncle. As he was already over 6 feet tall, we were reassured that he had not missed his growth potential. They met several times with our family therapist, but finally had to decide that he would pack a suitcase with some things he could eat in an emergency, because, even though he was very motivated, he simply could not bring himself to branch out. He was disappointed that I could not magically cure him, but relieved to be told he was otherwise "just fine."

Some children who eat a narrow range of foods do not grow normally, however, and that very small group will have one of two conditions: Restrictive eating (a rare condition I have not seen) or selective eating with such dysfunctional family dynamics that the young person has begun to refuse food out of distress and prefers to face hunger rather than give in to an intrusive parent. I must refer the reader to Bryan Lask and Rachel Bryant-Waugh's excellent discussion of restrictive eating in their book [68].

For selective eating aggravated by poor family interaction we would have weekly family therapy as the most urgent intervention, possibly art therapy as a useful form of individual expression for the child, and somewhat closer monitoring by our doctors for a return to adequate weight and growth. In rare cases where the child is actually failing to thrive, it might be necessary to begin the feeding and confirm the diagnosis in the  hospital or in the DTU.

# 4.4   Food phobia/functional dysphagia

We see about half a dozen children with food phobia a year. This is a frightening condition, and every time we hospitalize such a child, I wonder, "Is this going to be the one we can't help?" By the time children with this diagnosis are referred to us, they are invariably failing to thrive, often dehydrated, and losing weight. Food phobia is the sudden onset of refusal to eat or swallow. In its most severe form it may include all liquids, including the patient's own saliva, which is then continuously spit out. Food phobia is often preceded by a traumatic event: Choking, vomiting, or observing someone else doing so, but sometimes it is merely the unexplained onset of the *fear* of choking or vomiting. I can imagine that such phobias could be preceded by sexual trauma, but I have not seen this.

Because food phobia can be treated very effectively and because we have developed a protocol for doing so, I have created a separate chapter for this diagnostic entity (see Chapter 16).

# 4.5   Dieting gone awry: Imitative forms

A common referral to our clinic from community pediatricians is what we refer to as an appointment to "rule out eating disorder." Whenever we do not think a child referred to us actually has an eating disorder, we send them back to the referring doctor with the recommendation to look elsewhere for a diagnosis for their weight loss. But sometimes this kind of diagnosis is not so clear-cut.

It should not be surprising that with the pressure on women of all ages to be thin, some patients who do not have the actual brain disorder we call anorexia nervosa are tempted to engage in restrictive eating otherwise known as dieting. Add to that the encouragement to exercise and you have the young patient who loses a lot of weight and resists changing her behavior because of the positive social response to weight loss. Girls who were formerly not thin suddenly find boys paying attention to them. They now belong to the "thin girls" at school. Such patients may have the mild body image dissatisfaction of the normal American female, but are missing the delusional belief in themselves as fat that is the hallmark of full-blown anorexia nervosa. They are able to perceive themselves as thin and, by God, they want to stay that way. As such patients are still children, they cannot be expected to think like middle-aged adults; hence they are not as impressed as we are by the medical consequences of their behavior. They are, however, impressed by the consequences to their social life of hospitalization and tedious and time-consuming outpatient follow-up. This is their major disincentive to continued dieting. Yet, make no mistake, their concerns are real. We treat such patients initially as if they had anorexia because it is only "longitudinal experience" with such children on the part of the whole team that makes the actual diagnosis and can help the child understand how counterproductive this dieting behavior is *for their own goals.* It is perhaps these patients, whom one hears talking about how their eating disorder was "all about controlling what went into their mouth," who achieve a rapid "cure," gain some notoriety among their peers for having "given up anorexia," and become mini-experts on the condition. This disorder—"dieting gone awry"—bears little resemblance in the end to the miserable, chronic, and dangerous disease that is true anorexia nervosa.

How do you sort this out in a general practice? I don't believe you can. Let the experienced eating-disorder team tackle this one.

When they are "cured," they will be returned to their pediatric provider, as long-term eating-disorder follow-up is rarely indicated.

There is also a subgroup of children with severe emotional/psychological disorders whose distress manifests as true lack of appetite. Unlike young people with anorexia nervosa they do not have constant food thoughts (until they are starved enough), and they do not have the delusional belief in their own fatness. They usually will eat things that no person with restricting anorexia would touch, such as high-fat items; they just eat small amounts of whatever they eat or sometimes refuse to eat at all. Differentiating this from anorexia nervosa is complex and best left to the multidisciplinary eating-disorder team, unless you have a very experienced child psychologist and a physician willing to do very close follow-up.

# 5 It is not the parents' fault

If you have been to our website at www.kartiniclinic.com, or spoken to us at all, then you have heard us say it: We treat children with eating disorders in the belief that *parents do not cause and children do not choose to have eating disorders.* Let me say it again: Parents do not cause eating disorders.

I could end the chapter here, but because this has been one of the most pernicious and pervasive myths about anorexia nervosa to follow us out of the last century, I will discuss it a bit further. Jim Locke, child psychiatrist at Stanford University, relates in his introduction to Laura Collins' book *Eating with Your Anorexic*: "I had been taught that adolescents with eating disorders were likely victims of parents over controlling them and that the only avenue left to them to experience independence was through food and weight" [74]. Dr. Locke was not the only psychiatrist, fairly recently trained, to receive this teaching as the gospel; it is still recited to us by many psychiatrists and therapists, and not just about childhood anorexia either. Bruno Bettelheim, famed child psychologist, was crystal clear in his belief that mothers were responsible for the sad condition(s) we call autism. And in one fell swoop this outdated (and incorrect) theory alienated and cut off the very people who could help.

Parents—especially mothers—feel guilty whenever anything goes wrong with their children. As parents, we feel that we should be able to protect our children from all misfortune, and that if we can't, we must have somehow neglected to do something. I am told by my colleagues who are cancer doctors that parents of children with cancer often feel this way as well: "What did I do wrong? Should we have had the basement tested for radon? Should we have moved out of the city? Away from the radio towers?" and so on.

When I tell parents for the first time that their child's anorexia is not their fault, they almost always cry, even fathers. But then an odd transformation takes place: They begin to argue with each other or with me. If they are divorced, the parent least in favor of the divorce may want the illness to have been about that. In their sadness and fear they may try to blame each other. If one parent has a drug or alcohol problem, the other may want to blame the child's illness on that. If the parents fight a lot, if the mother diets, if the father is a marathon runner and too-busy executive, they seek for the cause of their child's illness there. I have to then explain, "Sorry, folks, perhaps these things have caused other problems for you, but they did not cause this. Now it is up to us to make sure these problems don't interfere with getting and sustaining treatment for your child."

Sometimes, after a few weeks or months of working on their child's illness, after the initial relief they feel at not being blamed, parents begin to waver: "I disagree—I think we did cause this."

Now, why on earth would they want to believe this? I think it is because we humans hate the feeling of powerlessness more than anything. Rather than face the fact that random blows of fate can happen to our children despite us, we would rather take the blame for them. Inherent in accepting that we are to blame is the promise that if we just do things differently, we can somehow alter the outcome or prevent it from happening again.

What makes me so sure that parents don't cause this? The fact is that we have every kind of family and every kind of parenting in our clinic: Two-parent, traditional, strict, not strict, religious, atheistic, bohemian, single-parent, two-mother, two-father, grandparent—you name it, we've had it. There's a lot of bad parenting out there compared with the number of children with anorexia nervosa. And how about adult-onset AN? Whose "fault" is that? Do we continue to blame parents into middle age and older? Genetic studies of the role of family environment on who we are and what we suffer from have consistently shown that the effects of our genetic makeup become stronger as we grow older and the effect of shared family environment (parenting a prominent feature of this) becomes weaker. The reason our parents continue to "haunt us" as adults is not because of unresolved childhood issues, but because the older we get the more we resemble our closest genetic relatives, *whether or not we were raised by them* [94].

Even among those who work on behalf of families, some authors are not entirely clear on this subject. My, how hard parent blaming is to kill! At best, many practitioners give lip service to "parents don't cause," while secretly entertaining ambivalence. Take the newest "Position Paper" from the Academy of Eating Disorders published by authors I admire:

"It is the position of the Academy of Eating Disorders (AED) that whereas family factors can play a role in the genesis and maintenance of eating disorders, current knowledge refutes the idea that they are either the exclusive or even the primary mechanisms that underlie risk. Thus, the AED stands firmly against any etiologic model of eating disorders in which family influences are seen as the primary cause of anorexia nervosa or bulimia nervosa and condemns generalizing statements that imply families are to blame for their child's illness" [70].

Why not just stick to the last phrase condemning such statements? If families are not the primary cause, are they then to be understood to be a secondary or contributing cause? What does this mean? It sounds like an ambivalence to me.

What clinical difference does it make to accept that parents do not cause anorexia nervosa? Significant difference. We involve the parents from the first hour of treatment even in the treatment of young adults. Anorexia nervosa is a brain disorder, and even if a child were "old enough" to make decisions about their care, it is the brain that is impacted both by the disorder and the consequent starvation. Parents and physicians will need to be in charge of decision-making. My experience is that this is often met with relief on the part of the child. They are relieved that the adults are going to take charge of the illness they often recognize as out of control. Someone is going to keep them safe. We explain to parents and children that in our clinic we believe that in the home, the parents should be in charge. We hold parents responsible for making the living and paying the mortgage, and we hold them responsible for feeding their children. This means that adults will do the shopping, planning, and cooking because such duties are not part of the developmental goals of adolescence, and even if they were, children with anorexia nervosa simply cannot self-regulate around food. Period. If the parents are unwilling or unable to cook for their children and to eat with them, we have to tell them we cannot help them.

In our country, the admonishment to cook for our children (as opposed to reheating fast or pre-prepared food) runs into an astonishing amount of resistance, a challenge largely not shared by our colleagues overseas [89], even our nearest relatives in Australia, the United Kingdom, or Western Europe, where mothers still tend to cook. Apparently many of us are now too busy to do so. Parents are too busy, and they allow their children to be too busy to eat at home. All sports events and practices take place over the dinner hour, PTA meetings and board meetings also happen at these times, parents themselves go to the gym at dinnertime, and so on. Many people do not dare to eat later in the evening, because they think it will make them fat. I often point out that the Spanish, the Italians, and the French all eat much later than we do, and yet they are slimmer. At Kartini Clinic, we preach cooking and eating at home in a spirit of love, often to no avail. Even non-working parents are often resistant to cooking dinner every night.

Many families do have two parents who work outside the home, but that is not the real problem: Generations of women worked in the fields or factory and still managed to put dinner on the table and eat it with their children. In earlier times it was simply expected of mothers, and now it is no longer expected of either parent. But the Kartini Clinic expects it! We will not treat a child unless the parents both agree to this critical intervention.

# 5.1 Children do not choose to have anorexia nervosa

"Why are you doing this?" "Don't you know what you are doing to your family?" "How can you ruin your health like this?" "Aren't you afraid your teeth will erode away?" "Your bones break?" "Your heart stop?" In sheer frustration these are some of the many questions thrown at patients with anorexia nervosa. Imagine a child with leukemia or diabetes facing such accusations. Ask it often enough and the child believes it, too, especially our patients who tend to be overly conscientious and reluctant to be a burden.

The media is full of reports of former sufferers who "explain" why they "chose" anorexia to "deal with problems they didn't want to face." This is about as reliable as the twelfth-century leper explaining that he got leprosy because he committed adultery, but people are astonishingly willing to credit it.

I find the implication that our patients are responsible for their anorexia nervosa because they want to look like some famously starved model insulting and trivializing of their illness. As one 17-year-old patient of mine put it so well after she had had to stay back in school a year because of her hospitalizations, after her teeth were capped and her parents' bank account was drained, "Who would choose this loser disease? I would give anything never to have had it." The media reports only those fashion models who become famous for their lean lines, those girls who, formerly plump, now become most popular. They rarely report on the straight-A student who finally got into Stanford only to be asked to leave in her freshman year because her eating disorder cycled out of control; or the young marriages dissolved by a disease that consumes all your time and energy and depletes your sexual drive; or the athlete who is constantly "benched" for stress fractures that never quite heal. Who would choose it indeed?

Let us render the present chapter short and sweet: *We treat eating disorders in children in the belief that parents do not cause them and children do not choose to have them.*

# 6 When insurance refuses to pay

This chapter would not have been necessary if health insurance in the United States had unquestioned, enforced parity between mental health coverage and medical health coverage.

We all agree that the artificial separation of brain and mind, of physical and mental health, is just that: Artificial. But health insurance companies, until forced to by legislation, will continue to insure people differently for conditions they consider "mental."

A typical health insurance plan has very deep pockets on the medical side to help protect people financially from catastrophic and expensive illnesses. Mental health coverage, however, is usually scanty if present at all, and once it is used up, the patient has to pay privately for whatever care they or their children need. A standard policy might, for example, agree to pay for 20 mental health visits in two years and specifically exclude family therapy of any kind (interesting in this era of political focus on the family). At the insurance company non-physicians may be making decisions about whether treatment should be paid for and whether or not it is indicated. Sub-specialists know that their patient's care will not be reviewed by an equivalent sub-specialist even when it is reviewed by a doctor. In the field of eating disorders the insurance medical directors we get assigned to are often psychiatrists. They vary greatly in their orientation towards eating disorders, and it is rare that they have experience with young children. I have been told by some that it is clear that "the family is causing this mental illness" (anorexia) and that they will authorize only psychiatric care. I have even been told by non-psychiatrists that no part of the medical care will be authorized unless a psychiatrist does it, even those things clearly outside the usual scope of practice for psychiatrists, such as the treatment of starvation and bradycardia (low heart rate).

Some years ago I had a patient of modest means from rural Idaho whose parents flew to Portland to seek help for their starved 13-year-old daughter, because none was available where they lived. The mother quit her job and stayed in Portland for two months through a grueling inpatient and day hospital stay. Once their daughter was discharged, the parents flew from Idaho to Portland every week for months at their own expense until she was stable enough to be at home without direct follow-up. She did very well for half a year, until her first major relapse. Initially, when they first noticed a return of their daughter's almost extinguished eating-disordered behaviors, her parents still hoped they could handle it at home. They felt they could not face having to return to Oregon so far away. When they finally did contact us, she had already lost 14 pounds and needed to be re-hospitalized. Their nightmare started all over, this time with one cruel twist: The case manager at their insurance company now refused to authorize payment for the second hospitalization. I was told that the relapse was "clearly the parents' fault" and that if they had just known "how to comply" and how to "handle their spoiled daughter," she would not have needed further care. Incredibly, this manager had the power to refuse authorization. People who go to work every day, who pay their insurance premiums on time, were left to fend for themselves for the thousands of dollars her treatment cost.

At that time almost all insurance companies refused to pay anything for medical care of eating disordered children and although some companies still refuse today, this is no longer the norm. What changed?

In the early to mid-1990s the Eating Disorder Service at Stanford University, under Professor Iris Litt, piloted a very powerful insurance coding change with far-reaching consequences for children with eating disorders. The Stanford team began insisting that children be hospitalized only under certain conditions of medical compromise, and they coded their hospitalization accordingly. Compromised children were not being put in the hospital for "anorexia nervosa;" they were being put in the hospital for a set of carefully defined medical instability criteria: "Bradycardia," "orthostasis," "hypophosphatemia," "hypokalemia," and so on, as discussed in other chapters. This fit the insurance company's paradigm; it worked. Under Stanford's new system, only once the patient was medically stable (per strict criteria) were they discharged to outpatient care. I carried the Stanford approach home with me after a visit in 1998, determined to get services for ill children and adolescents in the Pacific Northwest.

I was met with a great deal of resistance. The insurance companies, not used to this approach, were very resistant to paying for care for eating-disordered patients out of the "medical bucket." I spent countless hours arguing with medical directors, who were not only reluctant to see pediatric anorexia nervosa as a "medical condition," but also reluctant to talk to me because I am not a psychiatrist. Oddly, some pediatric cardiologists, seeing these children on the general school-aged floor, on constant cardiac monitoring (telemetry) argued that their bradycardia was "because they were athletes," and no number of attempts to explain the programmatic necessity for such criteria convinced them otherwise.

I tried to explain to them that, like the well-known Jones Criteria for rheumatic fever, individual medical instability criteria such as bradycardia might have limited meaning, but that in combination, in the setting of semi-starvation, they were ominous. Psychiatric staff on the locked child/adolescent wards, although not really wanting to care for severely medically compromised patients, were nonetheless uncomfortable with and critical of this "medical approach" to what they viewed as a "psychological problem," one "caused by the family."

I argued that our patients were in the same position as a patient who is severely depressed, who cannot get care for his depression because of his limited mental health coverage, and who then shoots himself in the head and winds up in the intensive care unit. No one seems to think that the subsequent plastic surgery, ventilator care, and rehab for such a patient should be classified as "mental health" care. Yet the overt medical conditions of our severely starved children were still treated as "psychological" and their families were denied coverage [109].

Over the years we have honed the definition of "medical instability" *as it pertains to these starved pediatric patients.* I modified Stanford's criteria slightly for our use, and Stanford modified their own over the years. In 2002 the American Academy of Pediatrics reinforced these criteria and lent them credibility by publishing standards for general use [54]. These standards, incidentally, can be used for treating starvation of any etiology. I have given advice on the acute re-feeding of children whose caretakers have withheld their food and of children with other underlying diseases (such as cancer) who are also cachetic (severely wasted). All resident pediatricians, internists, and family practitioners should have a good understanding of re-feeding and of the rationale for the criteria for medical instability in starved children.

I have gradually been able to convince the insurance companies we work with that we will put in the hospital only those children who meet these criteria and that, conversely, we will discharge them as soon as they no longer meet them. This compromise has made it possible for our patients with anorexia nervosa to get the treatment they need. It allows us to begin the induction of re-feeding while they are in the hospital, the place it is most likely to succeed safely. It is my hope that eating-disorder physicians in the future will be able to work together with health insurance professionals to assure a high quality of care for children with eating disorders and assure also that valuable resources are not being squandered.

In the chapter on inpatient stabilization, I cover the details of the hospitalization criteria. But I feel I need to say a word about their use in the children's hospital. In developing these criteria, especially those covering bradycardia and orthostasis, we are making no statements about these two conditions in any patients except those who are starved. Under other circumstances bradycardia, for instance, may have a completely different implication and other "cutoffs" would apply.

Curiously, some of the greatest resistance to our use of these criteria has come from an unexpected source: A few pediatric cardiologists. As discussed in chapter 2, I have had more than one patient told by the cardiologist that the reason their heart rate is so low is because they are athletic. They have further been told that they will lose their "conditioning" with bed rest.

A child is not an adult. The experience of adult athletes does not pertain to children, especially starved children, however athletic. A heart rate in the low to mid-40s, much less the 30s, is not normal for a child. If it were an effect of training, it would not go away when their diet was normalized. At our hospital we have never yet seen a child whose heart rate did not normalize with re-feeding. But some of our families have been very unhappy about our recommendation for hospitalization in their severely bradycardic child, because a "heart doctor" said the condition was normal for "athletes."

This difficulty was illustrated by the case of a 15-year-old boy on our service whose parents brought him to us after failing many attempts at home to induce him to eat enough for the amazing amount he was exercising every day. It was not a happy working relationship from the start. They did not like the hospital rules and thought exceptions should be made for their son; they did not approve of the white rice on the menu at one meal; they did not want us to use "any medication," and they resented having to meet with a family therapist. Their son was very bradycardic (low heart rate), something that gradually began to improve with nutrition, but they nonetheless demanded to see a cardiologist as we were "keeping him" in the hospital "for his heart." Normally an athletic boy, he had begun to exercise nearly every waking moment, and would exercise under the sheets when his nurses were not in the room. "Exercise relieves stress for him," his father insisted. It was hard to give him enough calories to cover his increased metabolic needs with re-feeding, never mind the surreptitious exercise, so we had to keep him at bed rest followed by graduated activity until he could gain weight. The cardiologist told his parents that he felt their son's heart rate in the low 40s was "normal for him" and that any amount of bed rest would make him worse. The boy had become very orthostatic with re-feeding, and the cardiologist suggested to the parents that our prescribed limited activity was probably making him "more orthostatic." This was the end of any modest working relationship with our team. One morning I was making rounds and standing outside the door to the patient's room, trying to explain to his angry parents why he had to use the wheelchair when his orthostatic pulse differential was 50 BPM. The boy crept to the door to listen. We heard a loud crash and rushed in; he had collapsed. Fortunately he was not severely injured. Yet despite this clear example of the consequence of orthostasis, his parents removed him from the hospital against medical advice, stating we did not understand that their child was "an athlete" and "not like the others."

I relate this story to alert other physicians and parents to how counterproductive it can be for one specialty to treat another's work with disrespect. I cannot imagine entering the room of a neurosurgery patient and subverting the recommendations of the neurosurgeon. I believe this kind of disconnect between the specialties has to do with a profound misunderstanding of and prejudice against patients with anorexia nervosa in particular and brain disorders (psychiatric illnesses) in general. It is my hope that in the future cardiology and adolescent medicine can work together to clear up some of the physiologic mysteries of starvation in children of whatever etiology. One thing is clear: Without these well-defined medical instability criteria it would not be possible to get insurance coverage for the care of children with eating disorders within the medical units of a children's hospital.

# 6.1　The cost of not referring

Pediatricians, nurse practitioners, family physicians, and internists take justifiable pride in not referring every single problem that comes their way, but rather trying to manage what they can within the generalist setting. They also see a lot of dieting, some of which may be a fad and some of which is anorexia nervosa.

Let's be clear: Anorexia nervosa of childhood is a malignant brain disorder. Any illness that carries with it a mortality of 10% is very severe. As I write this chapter, a 20-year-old patient of ours lies at home dying of malnutrition. We met her when she was 13. Her parents have withdrawn her from treatment with us many times; they and she are "tired of fighting." She weighs 54 pounds and is 5 feet 4 inches tall. She can hardly move from the couch to the bathroom, her kidneys are shutting down, her thighs are wasted to sticks the size of a thin person's wrist, her bony structure is clearly visible beneath her tautly pulled skin, and as she lies there, often too weak to continue speaking, her only question for visitors is this: *Do you think I look fat?*

The cost of not making a timely referral is not just this sad and dramatic dying, nor even the growth stunting, the brain stunting, or the social stunting, the ruined college career, infertility, and broken bones, not even all this: It is also financial. The following case illustrates the costs to everyone of a late referral.

AG was a 14-year-old girl from a medium-sized town whose pediatrician had been following her closely for what the doctor felt was "unintentional weight loss" over two months. When seen in July, she denied any bingeing or purging and said she "ate normally." Family history revealed "hypothyroidism" in the females on the father's side of the family, many of whom were overweight. AG's mother was quite concerned about the weight loss, however, and so the pediatrician sent the daughter for laboratory studies and was concerned to note the following:

1. Low TSH 0.47 (normal 0.7–6.4)

2. Low T3 78 ng/dl (normal 97–186 ng/dl)

3. Normal T4 of 1.1 ng/dl (normal 0.9–1.4 ng/dl)

4. A thyroid gland that felt normal but was perhaps on the large side

5. Secondary amenorrhea (no menstruation) for six months (negative pregnancy test)

6. 25 pounds weight loss over two months

7. Lots of "nervous energy"

8. Insomnia

9. Cold intolerance

10. Intermittent palpitations

11. Alternating constipation and diarrhea

12. Depression despite getting "all A's in school"

The pediatrician was concerned about this constellation of symptoms and lab values and decided to refer her to an endocrinologist for a thyroid evaluation. The endocrinologist thought that the "disconnect between the suppressed TSH, low T3, and normal T4" was concerning. She suggested the possibility of "subacute thyroiditis with an initial hyperthyroid phase from leak of pre-formed hormone followed by eventual trend toward hypothyroidism." Alternate explanations were "major depression, eating disorder, or growth hormone deficiency."

AG's exam at the endocrinologist's office was unremarkable except for the slightly enlarged thyroid gland. She had been growing along the 10th percentile for height and had moved from the 40th percentile for weight to the 3rd percentile; further tests were ordered, and she was started on a low dose of propranolol. A thyroid uptake and scan was done (which was normal).

Further labs showed the following: Electrolytes and liver enzymes were normal; CBC was normal; BUN, creatitine, calcium, total protein, albumin, and bilirubin were all normal. IGF-1 was low normal at 199 ng/ml (normal 199–658 ng/ml); TSI =100% (normal < 125%). Abnormal labs included a low glucose of 41 (65–99) mg/dl, alkaline phosphatase of 55 U/L, (60–350), and a low estradiol (female hormone).

Follow-up was scheduled with both the endocrinologist and the pediatrician. At that point AG weighed 87.6 pounds. Two days later her weight had dropped to 84 pounds and her heart rate was 49 BPM. The pediatrician asked her mother to take her to a nutritionist and a therapist the following week. By early September her heart rate was 42 BPM (despite coffee) her urine-specific gravity was 1.000 (much too dilute), and the endocrinologist ordered growth hormone studies (serum prolactin, cortisol stimulation test, ACTH levels, and arginine-GHRH) to follow up on the low IGF-1 level. To rule out global hypopituitary functioning (because of the low thyroid hormone, the low estradiol, LH and FSH and relative short stature) a karyotype (genetic study) was ordered, and an MRI of the brain. Endocrine follow-up was requested for three weeks later. By the end of September AG was considerably weaker, her heart rate in the pediatrician's office was 45 BPM, and neither the therapist (whom the child enjoyed talking to) nor the dietician (who recommended "more food") were able to reverse the weight decline. It was at this point that we were consulted. All of the above findings were consistent with restricting anorexia nervosa; indeed they were typical for it. An eating-disorder consultation may include an EKG and the doctors' time, but little else that is costly.

A minimal summary of the cost of this work-up (fortunately confined to an endocrinologist, but one that more commonly would have also included a cardiologist for the bradycardia) follows in the table below. By the time this goes to press, the costs will almost certainly have gone up.

| | |
|---|---|
| Estradiol | $165.85 |
| TSH | $102.95 |
| LH | $105.60 |
| FSH | $89.80 |
| T4 | $30.20 |
| T3 total | $89.80 |
| CBC | $26.25 |
| Comp panel (with LFTS and e'lytes) | $35.84 |
| Bhcg | $45.10 |
| TSIG | $340.20 |
| T4 free | $109.50 |
| Prolactin | $119.30 |
| Thyroid autoantibody | $125.90 |
| ACTH | $101.70 |
| Cortisol | $90.05 |
| Thyroid update and scan | $302.40 |
| Isotope (for scan) | $120.00 |
| Physician interpretation of scan | $150.00 |
| Karyotype (R/o Turners) | $250.00 |
| Cortisol stimulation test (x2) | $99.00 |
| Arginine-GHRH test | $85.00 |
| MRI head with/without contrast | $2,200.00 |
| Physician interpretation | $660.00 |
| TOTAL | $5,448.40 |

The total of $5,448.40 does not include the endocrinologist's "new patient charge" or follow-up visits. Nor does it include the cost of the nutritionist and therapist during a time when her worsening condition was not being addressed by these modalities.

The above case is one in which the constellation of symptoms typical for anorexia nervosa was interpreted as an endocrine problem. More commonly an eating-disordered patient is referred to a cardiologist for "fainting" or to a gastro-endocrinologist for "abdominal pain," "weight loss," "constipation," "poor appetite," and occasionally "vomiting."

A pediatric cardiology consult would be charged at the following rates:

| | |
|---|---|
| Office consultation | $531.00 |
| EKG and physician interpretation | $140.00 |
| Chest X-ray and interpretation | $130.00 |
| ECHO | $1,036.00 |
| TOTAL | $1,837.00 |

A total of $1,837.00 would be spent for a visit to address "fainting."

A pediatric gastroenterology work-up would cost roughly as follows:

| | |
|---|---|
| Upper GI endoscopy | $680.00 |
| Versed sedation | $50.00 |
| Lower GI endoscopy | $921.00 |
| Hemocult test | $10.00 |
| Office consultation | $350.00 |
| TOTAL: | $2,011.00 |

A total of $2,011.00 would be spent to address "abdominal pain," "weight loss," and so forth.

Of course the answer to a diagnostic dilemma is unknown, by definition, until the diagnosis is made, but this chapter is a plea to remember that "common things are common," and certainly nothing is cheaper than a good food history. Given the constellation of symptoms and findings listed above, please, doctors and parents: Keep an eating disorder very high on the list of possibilities for weight loss.

# 7 Are you telling me it's a brain disorder?

I don't know what anyone else's experience with the human brain was like in medical school, but mine was humbling. Each of us was privileged to be given a whole human brain to hold in our hands and to take apart. Under the direction of Dr. Heidrun Behrent, Professor at RWTH University in Aachen, we used a long flat knife to peel away hard-to-see "layers" in the pickled, somewhat stiff gray mass. She told us stories about function as we went. We were very impressed, but there was such a lot to know, and I was never particularly good at it. Like everyone else I had to memorize the cranial nerves and the rough parts of what was understood about the functional components of this supremely important organ. Once I had passed my exams, I immediately forgot a lot of it. Like all aspiring pediatricians I tried to force myself to do a reasonable neurological exam with every physical, but it wasn't until I began to work intensively with eating-disordered children that the brain came into real focus for me.

One day, my associate pediatrician told me she had noticed mild tongue deviation in a patient referred to us to "rule out an eating disorder" and so had ordered an MRI. I was in the office the next day and got the call from the radiologist: There was a brain stem tumor, which neurosurgeon did I want to work with, and when would I tell the parents? From that moment the twelveth cranial nerve was seared into my brain—such is the power of context.

The course of treatment for this patient was interesting in many ways (she is still alive, graduated from college, and doing well.) From the moment of her diagnosis as a patient with a brain tumor, everyone's attitude toward her changed. She had been in the hospital on the eating-disorder service being re-fed, and she suffered from cachexia (wasting), intermittent vomiting, and increasing social isolation. Because she was painfully shy and somewhat withdrawn and because they had to clean up after her vomitus, the nurses (at that point still untrained by us) treated her like an "anorexic," with more than a hint of frustration. The resident house staff and their attending physicians, convinced this was a psychosocial condition, were annoyed to have to follow her with us. They felt helpless to deal with these "psych" issues. But from the moment her tumor was confirmed, their interest was galvanized. Now they knew what to do, now they knew what to think: A brain tumor—now that was real medicine! And the nurses who had been frustrated and put off were filled with pity and compassion for a patient now known to have a "real disease."

This stigmatization of the field of eating disorders and the patients themselves has been painful. Even today I have to convince new house officers and attending physicians that our patients have a "real," not a volitional, disorder. It is all about the brain, I tell them, that organ that commands us all, and I challenge them to get up to date in neuroimaging and neurobiology.

One day I attended a medical case conference carrying a new book called *Neurobiology in the Treatment of Eating Disorders* and sat next to the woman neurosurgeon whom I most admire. She looked down at the book in surprise: "What does neurobiology have to do with eating disorders?" she asked.

Well, everything.

In *Principles of Neuroscience*, Dr. Eric Kandel says this about brain function:

> What we commonly call mind is a range of functions carried out by the brain. The action of the brain underlies not only relatively simple motor behaviors such as walking, breathing and smiling, but also elaborative affective and cognitive behaviors such as feeling, learning, thinking and composing a symphony. As a corollary, the disorders of affect (feeling) and cognition (thought) that characterize neurotic and psychotic illness can be seen as disturbances of brain function.

Kandel is a psychiatrist and neurobiologist at Columbia University who received the 2000 Nobel Prize in Medicine for his work with the human brain and discoveries concerning signal transduction in the nervous system. He goes on to point out that *"affective and character traits are also anatomically localized"* (my emphasis) [53, p. 5, 12].

When you think about it, how can it be otherwise? When did we come to treat the end product (behavior) of this powerful organ as if it were something emanating from the ether, not a result of physiology?

Kandel's medical textbook *Principles of Neural Science* discusses brain disorders such as schizophrenia, about which a bit more is known than about eating disorders, and his conclusions are thought-provoking. This discussion of schizophrenia we could easily substitute the words *anorexia nervosa* for *schizophrenia/(* and make perfect clinical and biological sense.

In the early history of psychiatry, Eugen Bleuler, Swiss psychiatrist and psychologist, born April 30, 1857, proposed that schizophrenia "reflected not a single entity but a group of closely related illnesses characterized by disorder of thought rather than dementia (intellect)" [53, p. 855].

The various clinical forms of anorexia—restricting, binge purging, and so-called EDNOS—have strong common threads, but I think they similarly are likely to represent a group of closely related illnesses rather than just one. Anyone who has treated children with anorexia nervosa will tell you that their intellectual functioning is intact (provided they are not too starved), although they are suffering from a seemingly intractable disorder of thought. They too suffer from a form of "failure of reality testing," being unable to examine their beliefs and perceptions realistically and to compare them to what actually is happening in the world. Those of my pitifully thin patients who will not swallow a penicillin tablet for strep throat because of the delusional belief that the calories they contain (perhaps 1 or 2) will push them over the edge "into (even greater) obesity," as they believe, fit this description, usually applied only to schizophrenia. I believe that this implacable perception of themselves as fat is a form of hallucination (abnormal perception) and delusion (aberrant belief). No doubt this is why many of our patients respond to the use of low doses of the same antipsychotics used to treat schizophrenia. This will be discussed later under medical stabilization and in Dr. Desocio's chapter on psychopharmacology.

Going even further to dissect out brain disorders from their former matrix of purely psychosocial etiology, Kandel reports, as we did in chapter 5 ("Genetics of Eating Disorders") that, unlike conditions inherited via simple Mendelian processes, schizophrenia is a multifactorial, polygenic disease "like diabetes and hypertension" that likely "require(s) the accumulation of several genetic defects as well as environmental factors" [53, p. 857].

Explaining the differences observed among patients with schizophrenia he writes something that I wish could be branded into our pediatric and adolescent medicine texts as it so easily could have been written about anorexia nervosa: "[E]ven though all people who have schizophrenia (or any other mental illness) are similar in important ways and all will, by definition, share the *defining* features of the disease, different individuals suffering from schizophrenia will nevertheless differ in distinctive ways that may influence the course of the disease, even its outcome" [53, p. 867].

# 7.1 Neuroimaging

Neuroimaging has brought us a few tentative steps closer to localizing anorexia nervosa (AN) among the trillions of neurons we possess. It is unlikely that there is one area solely responsible for either the vulnerability of certain genetically predisposed individuals or for the panoply of symptoms most patients report, and indeed recent magnetic resonance spectroscopy (MRS) studies have implicated the cingulate, frontal, temporal, and parietal regions in AN [30]. Additionally it has long been known that gray and white matter both shrink in AN, something that may not entirely remit.

Bulimia nervosa (BN) has been studied as well and may lend insights into both conditions, as people with BN are of normal weight, allowing us to begin to sort pure starvation effects from those changes that may be characteristic of the actual brain disorder(s). University of Cambridge scientists E. A. Stamatakis and M. M. Hetherington report the following:

Typically, anorexia nervosa (AN) is associated with cerebral spinal fluid spaces enlargement which generally recover as a function of re-feeding. However,

specific cortical areas fail to correct in weight restored
anorectic patients suggesting trait-related abnormalities. Functional changes in AN associated with starvation reverse with weight recovery, however, reduced
5-HT2A receptor binding may be fundamental to the
pathophysiology of AN since this remains after long
term weight restoration. Structural studies of bulimia
nervosa (BN) provide evidence of brain atrophy, in the
absence of significant weight loss but potentially related
to chronic dietary restriction. Functional investigations
reveal reduced thalamic and hypothalamic serotonin
transporter availability in BN which increases with
longer illness duration. Thus, BN is associated with
substantial structural and functional alterations despite normal weight. Recent advances in neuroimaging
techniques and their interpretation are increasing our
understanding of normal processes in the control of food
intake including neuroanatomical correlates of hunger
and satiety. Taken together with the structural and
functional changes observed in the ED, neuroimaging
provides a powerful platform to identify the underlying trait-related pathophysiological mechanisms in the
aetiology and maintenance of AN and BN [116].

How are we to put this all together? Is the picture we are
building specific to anorexia nervosa and other eating disorders,
or is it a generalized picture of "how things go wrong" in the
human brain? As we begin to localize specific disorders to their
"home bases" and "major transit centers," we see that most illnesses can be referred to anatomic sites, some of which overlap.
Thus Parkinson's disease is known to affect the basal ganglia and

schizophrenia possibly to affect the thalamus [33] and nucleus accumbens [49], striatum, and superior temporal cortex. According to D. C. Jimerson, MD, professor of psychiatry at Harvard Medical School and B. Wolfe, PhD [51], RN, patients with bulimia nervosa show impaired post-ingestive satiety and blunted plasma cholecystokinin responses. Signals from the periphery (gut, pancreas, abdominal skin, etc.), including gut-related peptides and the adipokines, interact with hypothalamic peptides in the regulation of feeding and body weight.

Without doubt the explosion in the technology of brain imaging will bring us a flood of new information about what is going on with anorexia nervosa and where. But what will this mean for those of us who are clinicians and for parents worried about their individual child?

Even without sophisticated imaging we need to be aware that it is the physical brain we are dealing with. We need to share this *de-stigmatizing* point of view with our patients and families. Whenever I meet a patient for the first time and begin their physical exam, I start by saying: "I am going to do your exam today. It will not include needles or blood drawing, and there will be no pelvic exam. In this clinic we are most interested in the brain." They often seem surprised. What did they think I was going to be interested in? Then I lay out my simple instruments, including a small vial of oil of eucalyptus to test the first cranial nerve, and I explain every step of the way what I am doing. My message: You are not just an eating disorder to me—not an "anorexic" or a "bulimic" but a person whose family has become so concerned about your health that they have asked me to take a look at you, to listen to you, and to find out what I think may be going on. And the thoughts and feelings that have caused you so much confusion and pain are not your fault. Together we will listen to your brain and find out how to proceed.

# 8 What heritability means and what it does not

What does it mean to say that something is inherited? It seems fairly clear in the case of eye color or wrinkled versus smooth skin on a pea. But today many human traits under study appear not to follow simple Mendelian rules for heritability. Partly this may be because of the complex nature of what we choose to study, such as violent behavior, depression, or anxiety. These things that seem so clear when we talk about them may actually be aggregates of many things, some more important than others. And what fuels a certain behavior may not be a single thing, but many things, the presence of any one of which may be necessary but not sufficient to "cause" or "explain" complex traits, especially behavioral ones.

I am not a geneticist, which may turn out to be helpful to those of you reading this who wish to hear about the genetics of anorexia nervosa laid out in plain English.

Family and twin studies have reinforced the observation that anorexia nervosa and bulimia nervosa have a strong genetic component [13] [56]. The heritability of anorexia nervosa is reported to lie somewhere around 70% [6] [121]. Does this mean that you have a 70% chance of getting it if another family member has it? Or that 70% of people with a family history of AN will get it? *It means neither of those things.* The heritability of a trait tells us the relative contributions of genes and the environment in a population; it is not a statement about any one individual.

Heritability can be roughly estimated by looking at the rate at which a given trait occurs in identical twins minus the rate at which it occurs in non-identical twins, times two (we each have two sets of chromosomes). Or perhaps more clearly, it means that 70% of the variation you see in the trait (variation in the phenotype) is attributable to genetics (variation in the genotype) and the rest (30%) is attributable to the environment [66].

You might say, "So 30% of what I see in this disease called anorexia nervosa is attributable to the environment," but actually it's a shade more complex than that. Geneticists divide the "environment" into two types: "Shared environment" (such as the effects of being raised in the same family) and "nonshared environment" (such as one twin marrying a man who then takes her to his country which is at war and the other marrying a local man and staying home in a peaceful land). Curiously and entirely counter-intuitively, for those of us who are parents and who spend a great deal of time worrying about the effect of our parenting on our children, *for most behavioral traits that have been studied, the effect of shared environment appears to be small. Most of the effect comes from nonshared environment* [100]!

And there's one more twist: Non-shared environment is itself powerfully affected by genetics. For example, not many people injure themselves bungee jumping. Why? Those who bungee-jump tend to be risk-takers with an established safety strategy. Is risk-taking behavior inherited [108]? It is. Just ask any grandmother or parent of more than one: Some of us are timid, some are brave, wild, and crazy, and most of us are somewhere in between, but these traits are present since our early years and are very resistant to change. It has become increasingly clear that the boundary between genetics and environment is more apparent than real: A reciprocal interaction between the two is almost certainly the norm. After all, people select many aspects of their lifestyle (their environment) partly for genetic reasons, and the same environmental stressors affect different people differently, based on their individual genetic susceptibility to such stressors. This is the origin of the common observation that there are people for whom the "glass is always half empty" or "always half full."

These observations must not lead us to think that one style of person/environment interaction happens in superior individuals and the other in inferior ones, rather that we all interact with our environment, at all times, based on who we are genetically and who we have become through a lifetime of environmental interactions.

Gorwood *et al.*, in their article "Human Genetics in Anorexia Nervosa," put it more clearly still:

> Anorexia nervosa is a severe eating disorder characterized by restricted eating, the relentless pursuit of thinness and obsessive fears of being fat. The involved risk factors are probably numerous, but the existence of a genetic vulnerability has been proposed for decades. The heritability in the broad sense is computed on the basis of aggregation studies, treated twin samples and twin studies from the general population. Many difficulties make this heritability estimation problematic, but the convergence of the results (from family studies and two types of twin studies) gives the most convincing evidence in favor of a major role of genetics in the vulnerability to anorexia nervosa, with a heritability around 70%. Regarding the analysis of candidate genes, the most frequently studied is the 5-HT(2A) gene, with positive and negative results [41].

In her article on contemporary thinking about the role of genes and environment in eating disorders, Cynthia Bulik reports, "Relatives of individuals with eating disorders have approximately a tenfold greater lifetime risk of having the disorders than relatives of unaffected individuals" [13].

Several studies hoping to locate a candidate gene for anorexia nervosa are under way [42] [7]. And studies are likewise being undertaken to discover the role genes play in bulimia nervosa [14], selective eating, binge eating, body dysmorphism, and even low self-esteem. And if you doubt that any of these things run in families, for whatever reason, you have not taken enough family histories!

An example I often use to explain how the environment and genetics might interact in anorexia nervosa is that of type 1 diabetes (IDDM), the kind that affects children and requires insulin. In former times mothers were blamed for this disease, too. People thought that if your child got type 1 diabetes, it meant that you fed them too much sugar. We now think that to get IDDM you have to carry the genes that predispose you and make you vulnerable to attack from an environmental trigger. In the case of IDDM this "trigger," this "environmental stressor," may well be a virus that initiates an autoimmune cascade whose target organ are certain cells in the pancreas. Even after millions of dollars spent in research and the best scientific efforts, we still cannot reach inside a child and "turn off" diabetes, but we can keep the disease from destroying the child by controlling insulin, diet, and exercise. It's not easy, but it can be done. I propose that children with anorexia nervosa have a genetic vulnerability to this disorder and that something in the environment triggers an (autoimmune?) cascade whose target organs are certain cells in the brain. No therapist, no matter how talented, can reach inside a person and turn off anorexia nervosa either, but again, we can keep the disease from destroying the child by controlling diet and exercise while therapeutic interventions promote brain healing and learning.

What is the trigger to developing anorexia nervosa (AN)? Quite simply, we do not know. In fact, we have no idea. I am concerned that despite the universe of possibilities, we have been so constrained by old prejudices that we continue to exert all our effort looking in one arena only (the psychosocial) for the answer. I propose that we expand our search to the biological. A trigger could as easily be a virus as it could be a psychological stressor or a diet. Viruses are environmental stressors to living organisms. Only further research will tell about the cause of AN.

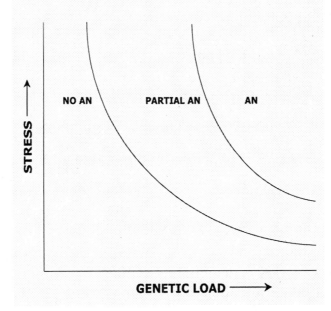

**Figure 8.1:** A rough estimate of the effect of environmental factors and genetic predisposition on eating-disorder development. (My own conceptualization.)

In figure 8.1, I have attempted to show how environmental triggers (of yet unknown kind) could interact at a given level of genetic "load" or predisposition to produce either subclinical eating-disorder symptoms, "partial AN," or even full-blown AN; implicit in the figure is the conclusion that at a very low level of genetic load (or none) no amount of stress will produce AN or even partial AN, though it may produce other, unspecified problems.

In her excellent book *Eating Disorders: A Clinical Guide to Counseling and Treatment*, Monika Woolsey, MS, RD, offers three insights from an experienced dietician's point of view:

- Eating-disordered individuals have a high incidence of functional disruption along the anterior pituitary axes, further supporting the theory that disruption of neurotransmitter production and maintenance is an important first step in the development of anorexia, bulimia, and binge-eating disorder.

- Some of the first symptoms of these disorders that are apparent externally are changes in behavior and mood, but treatment of the individual with these diseases requires medical as well as psychological intervention.

- Physiological changes along the hypothalamic-pituitary axes often exist for months after weight gain or stabilization is achieved. Though weight gain is an indicator of the direction of progress, it is not the bottom line [129].

What does this understanding of the genetic contribution to AN mean for the care of children and youth with this disease? It means that we have to rethink how we approach what we see in families. Not infrequently a mother or father brings their child to us with clear anorexia nervosa, but during the course of our extensive interviews we discover that one (or both) parent has major eating issues, if not a frank eating disorder, or that although no one in the family seems to have an eating disorder as such, they do have a strong history of anxieties and even phobias (like the patient whose aunt was so germ phobic she showed up at a family funeral wearing a baseball glove). Should we be surprised? With a heritability of 70%? The daughter resembles her affected parent not because her parent has somehow "influenced her in a bad way," but because daughter and parent share roughly half their genes.

And there are other more subtle effects which contribute to this picture if you delve deeply enough into people's life stories. For example, many people with AN are high-achieving and perfectionistic. Because we often choose a mate compatible with our expressed traits, it would not be unusual for such a woman to marry a man who is himself successful and high-achieving (there is less longitudinal movement among the socioeconomic classes than you might hope), with a job that rewards single-mindedness and perseverance. Now the daughter has a "double dose" of traits known to be associated with AN [12].

In the course of treating a child like this we have to focus on two things: 1) Helping defuse any belief the family may have that either parent "did this" to their child and 2) helping the parents understand that they, too, may have behaviors or conditions that need attention if their child is to get well. Sound complex? It is the essence of complexity and the reason treatment requires a whole team.

The fact that you are likely to run into more than one affected family member has implications for treatment and prognosis, just as it does for all conditions with a strong genetic (or perhaps epigenetic!) underpinning. The affected family member may or may not be diagnosed, and they may or may not be willing to get treatment. In the case of a brain disorder like anorexia nervosa or bulimia nervosa the affected parent may very well be resistant to change, as resistant as their child is. At the Kartini Clinic we tell parents in our parent group that if a patient's parent is known to be active in their own eating disorder and refuses to get help, our experience has been that the child's own prognosis is very poor. If our treatment team is convinced that one (or both) of the parents has an eating disorder, we must insist that they seek treatment. If they will not, we explain why we can't help them. Often parents will do for their child what they would not have done just for themselves.

Why does it matter so much if the parent is eating disordered? We have had a lot of experience with this: Not only might the parent's eating-disordered behaviors (restricting, "dieting," even purging) be triggering for the child, but invariably as the child's weight goes up, the parent becomes anxious that we are "going to make the child too heavy." The moment the child senses this, we have lost the battle. They will not have confidence in their treatment team and will be resistant to further weight restoration.

Placing emphasis on the genetic contribution to eating disorders is not a subtle way of blaming the parents. It is a way of freeing them from guilt and should be emphasized in this light. Presented appropriately, it can be powerfully de-stigmatizing.

Several studies are under way to pinpoint the genetic variants that predispose a person to anorexia nervosa, but not only are such variants still unknown, the relevant environmental triggers are still entirely unknown and may not even be psychological.

## Clinical pearls

- The heritability of anorexia nervosa is somewhere around 70%.

- This does *not* mean that if a relative has it, their children must necessarily have it.

- If a first-degree relative of yours has it, your risk of getting it is about ten times that of the general population.

- Shared environment plays only a modest role.

# 9 What happens when my child won't eat?

A solid understanding of the effects of starvation in humans is essential for any physician who cares for patients with anorexia nervosa and other wasting disorders of childhood and adolescence. One way to define true anorexia nervosa would be to subtract from the symptoms that our patients express those effects that can be universally ascribed to starvation itself and then see what we are left with. Could anorexia nervosa be a series of events, of whatever etiology, whose final common pathway is the starved state, events that are extinguished when we forcefully return the patient to a well-fed state? In other words, is re-feedin enough?

The following discussion of the starvation study done at the University of Minnesota during WWII is somewhat technical and detailed, but I have seen it referred to by a number of parents on online forums and discussions. They appear to have read it in some detail. I have yet to meet another doctor who has done so.

## 9.1 The Minnesota semi-starvation study

To begin to think about these questions, we need to review a seminally important study undertaken at the University of Minnesota, one that, due to today's increased restrictions on research with human subjects, will never be repeated. Additionally we will discuss what is known from periods of famine, especially famine during the most recent world wars. The horrors of starvation and death caused by World War II are appropriate to our discussion here: Let us never forget that human starvation *of whatever cause* is seriously harmful. This is every bit as true for patients with anorexia nervosa as it was for inmates of the concentration camps.

By 1944 it had become clear to the Allies fighting in both the European and the Pacific theaters that the war was creating a huge field of human starvation: Large populations of civilians were living under conditions that ranged from outright famine (in Holland) to chronic under-nutrition (in France), to say nothing of prisoners of war and inmates of the concentration camps, where starvation was but one of their problems. Further, once the war was over, it was clear that the Allies would have to take on the nutritional rehabilitation of large numbers of people, but little hard data was available on the effects of either starvation or re-feeding [59, p. xxiii].

Scattered clinical observations of starving people were being carried out at that time by doctors and researchers, some of whom were not only starving themselves, but eventually starved to death. Their field notes bear examining by those of us who care for eating-disordered children because of the remarkable similarities of their observations and ours: Starvation by famine, as by anorexia nervosa, was characterized by loss of weight, weakness, depression, polyuria (frequent urination), bradycardia (low heart rate), and increased relative hydration of the body [59, p. 14].

Treating reluctant patients with anorexia nervosa can be a challenge. We often ask ourselves what it is we are actually observing when we see our angry, often narcissistically self-involved, resentful patients. A few observations from wartime experience are relevant to this: "From the grumbling and grousing that are inevitably provoked when the energy intake is deficient to the extent of 15–20 percent, to the apathy and dissolution of higher human qualities that come with severe starvation, there is a wide variety of psychological reactions to hunger, many of which are almost, of themselves, diagnostic of the level of calorie intake" [59, p. xiii].

Apparently hunger itself unravels the normally empathetic, social personality. Equally interesting to the subject of reluctant acceptance of treatment, universally observed in patients with anorexia nervosa and perhaps wrongly attributed to the disorder itself, is the following observation on the process of bringing relief to starved people during a famine: "One of the curious, and rather disconcerting, psychological manifestations of starvation, seen repeatedly in Western Europe, was the unresponsive and uncooperative attitude of those to whom relief was brought. It disappeared without trace when calorie intakes rose above 1,500–1,800 a day" [59, p. xiv].

## Experimental design

To rapidly acquire the information the U.S. government needed to deal appropriately with the varied victims of starvation, the University of Minnesota, under the direction of Ancel Keys, undertook a large controlled experiment to study the effects of semi-starvation (goal weight loss of 25% of total body weight) on otherwise healthy men. Thirty-two young men, conscientious objectors to the war who volunteered to serve their country in this meaningful way, were recruited for study. These men, ranging from 20 to 33 years old, were subjected to an extensive battery of physical as well as psychological testing before being accepted, and then moved to residential housing at the university. For twelve weeks of a control period they were fed adequate calories of 3,492 kcals/day with 112 g protein, 124 g fat, and 482 g carbohydrates [59, p. 72] in order to *maintain* their healthy weight. Throughout the experiment they were expected to work at a job on campus for fifteen hours a week, walk twenty-two miles outdoors each week, and walk on a treadmill at 3.5 mph on a 10% grade for thirty minutes a week, in addition to walking to and from the dining hall, which added another two–three miles a week. This exercise regimen was strictly enforced until the latter half of the semi-starvation period, when weakness and apathy made it almost impossible. Interestingly, even then the men maintained their exercise protocol, but began to slack at their jobs. Additionally all thirty-two were expected to attend classes for twenty-five hours a week for a total of forty-eight hours per week occupation with the study, or the equivalent of a full-time job [59, p. 69].

The twelve-week control period was followed by twenty-four weeks of semi-starvation: Only two meals a day were served (at 8:30 AM and 5:00 PM), consisting of whole-wheat bread, potatoes, cereals, turnips, and cabbages—in other words, those foods available to the hungering people of Europe. There was very little animal protein and almost no fat in these rations, similar to the self-imposed diet of most of our patients with eating disorders. The nutritional breakdown for this twenty-four-week period of the study was 1,570 kcals consisting of about 50 g protein and 30 g fat [59, p. 74].

If 1,570 kcals/day seems draconian in a working person, please keep in mind that not only do many popular diets place clients on calorie levels like this or sometimes much lower, but our patients are nearly always discovered to be ingesting closer to 1,000 kcals/day or less, sometimes much less, with 0–15 g fat/day. Our patients achieve these numbers by assiduously avoiding all but fat-free milk products or drinking soy as a substitute, eating no meat, and avoiding all added sources of lipids.

The Minnesota Semi-Starvation Study (MSSS) was carefully controlled in all its aspects. Extensive physiological and psychological testing was undertaken at prescribed intervals under controlled conditions (e.g. air-conditioned rooms in the summer, after a meal). In order to achieve a weight loss of 25% in all subjects the food intake of each was calculated individually, as it was known that people lose weight at differing rates. Rations were therefore adjusted to keep the rate of weight loss steady and a total of no more than 25%.

Rehabilitation (re-feeding) was begun at the end of the twenty-four weeks of semi-starvation with a restricted diet for twelve weeks followed by another eight weeks of unrestricted (ad lib) re-feeding where the amount of food was not controlled but was measured and recorded.

## Consequences of starvation

All subjects in the study achieved the desired weight loss of 25%, with profound consequences to their health, both physically and psychologically, despite the fact that 25% is less than the weight loss achieved by many sufferers of AN.

So what constitutes severe weight loss? Even the parents of children who have been brought to me with weight losses from 25 to 30% of their usual weight are shocked to hear me refer to them as "starved." With premorbidly (before the illness) fat children, the parents often seem to recognize that their child is in trouble, but I have had more than one physician refer to an overweight child who has lost greater than 40% of their usual weight as "better off." Professor Keys tells us that "Most human beings can tolerate a weight loss of 5 to 10 percent with relatively little functional disorganization. At the other extreme, save for exceptional individuals, human beings do not survive weight losses greater than 35 to 40 percent" [59, p. 18]. Yet in his chapter on AN [59, p. 967] he mentions a 16-year-old patient who survives a weight loss of 47.5%, and most eating-disorder doctors have had patients with similar weight loss histories. Perhaps it is that our patients tend to suffer starvation in a setting of cleanliness, warmth, and good medical care, conditions not common during wartime or in detention camps. Furthermore, in the recent past (World War II), patients who were starved often died of tuberculosis, which is today an entirely treatable disease. In studying European children who had suffered from famine during and after World War I, decreases in body weight were found in the range of 25–40%. Ranges above this (closer to 50%) were found only in pediatric cadavers. Yet even much lower levels of weight loss than these which persist over time can interrupt normal childhood growth and development [59, p. 995-996].

What is the difference between *acute total fasting* and *prolonged semi-starvation*? Some children do not receive timely intervention because their parents and doctor tell themselves "she/he is still eating." In children with food phobia (see Chapter 3: "Eating Disorders of Childhood"), you might see acute food refusal over a period of many days, but in anorexia nervosa we typically see prolonged *semi-starvation* of one degree or another with some intake persisting. Keys reports three differences between the following states: 1) In acute total fasting the hunger sensation disappears after a few days, whereas in prolonged semi-starvation it is progressively accentuated, 2) Ketosis (where the body accumulates by-products of self-digestion) typically develops only in acute starvation, although we see it in anorexia nervosa when several meals have been completely skipped, i.e. in mini bouts of acute total fasting, and 3) Famine edema (where the body accumulates large amounts of fluid under the skin and in the abdomen) has not been reported in total starvation or fasting.

In the Minnesota study careful measurements done on these formerly healthy, now starved, young men showed several findings relevant to our patients and discussed below.

## Physiological consequences

**Fat mass:** Fat mass, which tended in the study to decrease more rapidly and more dramatically than other tissues, was shown to increase more rapidly than other tissue mass on re-feeding, with a clear tendency to the development of obesity with ungoverned dietary rehabilitation (i.e. "ad lib" eating [59, p. 126]). *This is a critically important observation with many ramifications for the outpatient care of our patients* and is discussed in depth in the chapters on outpatient care.

**Skeletal muscle mass:** Of 359 autopsies done on adults in the Warsaw Ghetto who died of starvation alone, only 2.7% had well-preserved muscle mass. Severe muscle wasting was reported for 61%. This is in strong contrast to the belief held by many of our patients (and some families and coaches) that weight loss will make them stronger and better athletes. The atrophy seen in striated muscle during the controlled MSSS is apparently also seen in smooth muscle, on autopsy [59, p. 186].

**Heart size in children:** The heart appears to diminish in size along with the body. Autopsies done on children who died of famine in Russia during World War I showed cardiac weights 20–40% or more below the normal average for their age, about the same percentage as of their total weight loss [59, p. 199]. Additionally, the heart in starvation was notable for its "softness, paleness and flabbiness" [59, p. 206]. Functional changes included bradycardia, low blood pressure, and syncope.

**Thyroid gland:** A decrease in thyroid activity has been reported for all periods of starvation studied. Myxedema (low thyroid induced edema) of hypothyroidism has been reported in famine so often that it is referred to as *Kriegsoedem* (war edema) by the Germans. It is very common for patients with anorexia nervosa to have low T4 or T3 level and sometimes low TSH (all are thyroid hormones) or their precursors without frank hypothyroidism: These abnormally low values normalize with re-feeding just as *Kriegsoedem* does.

**Pituitary gland:** The picture of starvation has often been described as one of pituitary atrophy [59, p. 214], with low levels of thyroid and sex hormones and pituitary underdevelopment seen at autopsy in men who starved to death.

**Bones:** Although no significant changes were noted in the MSSS subjects, more prolonged periods of semi-starvation (such as during wartime food shortages) have been shown to harm bone health. The effect of hypo-estrogenism and amenorrhea on the bones of young women is well known [80] [40], yet it was somewhat surprising to read of "hunger osteoporosis" in starved adults (famine) who had previously healthy bone mass and yet reported back pain and limb pain, with decreased bone density on X-ray as the only finding.

**Increased relative hydration:** Psychogenic polydipsia (over-drinking of water) was observed in the study participants (as we see it today in anorexia nervosa), with some men drinking fifteen cups of coffee a day. Even apart from this extreme ingestion, starvation is also well known to increase the relative hydration of

the whole body. Large amounts of water can be stored in the form
of obvious edema, as well as retained throughout many tissues in
a way that will not cause detectable edema of the skin. Diuresis
(copious urination) during re-feeding is therefore common.

## Psychological consequences

The above outlined physical findings are familiar to the eating-
disorder doctor, but what was seen psychologically in the Minnesota study? Where was the brain in all this?

After the second month of semi-starvation it became clear that
major psychological changes were taking place in the lives of these
formerly "normal" young men. Interviews with survivors of this
experiment report that, indeed, as far as they were concerned, the
major effects of starvation *were* psychological. I have reported their
observations below without comment, because I know that physicians who treat children with anorexia nervosa and those children's
parents who read this will recognize many of the observations and
may even smile at a few.

- The subjects became fixated on the timing of meals, not
  wanting to wait at all and were annoyed if meals were late.

- They made strange and distasteful concoctions of their food
  items with a huge increase in the use of condiments and salt.

- They toyed with their food, sometimes for hours.

- They smuggled food into their rooms (bunks) and consumed
  it privately.

- They dawdled for hours over a meal.

- They became obsessed with food, which became the principal subject of conversation.

- They fixated on any mention of food or eating in books they read or movies they watched.

- Cookbooks, menus, and information bulletins on food became intensely interesting to men who had never been interested in the subject before.

- They collected recipes.

- Some read food advertisements and tirelessly compared prices.

- One decided to go into agriculture to raise food, and several discussed becoming cooks.

- Toward the end of the starvation period a few subjects became annoyed with the "tyranny of food" and expressed disgust at other people's "animal interest" in the subject, even though many reported later that they felt vicarious pleasure from watching other people eat food or from merely smelling food.

- Several tried to suppress their interest in eating by vigorous and excessive gum chewing or smoking. In fact gum chewing became so excessive (up to forty packs a day) that it had to be severely limited.

- Excess coffee and tea drinking (fifteen cups a day) had to be controlled.

- They wanted their food always served as hot as possible.

- Once they reached the re-feeding stage, there was a marked deterioration in table manners.

- They began to spend more and more time alone, reporting it was "too tiring" to be around others.

- Their sense of humor disappeared.

- They were more irritable and egocentric, even though they previously had not been.

- They went on shopping outings and bought things that they later were puzzled to explain and regarded as "junk."

- Sexual interest was all but extinguished (testicular size is known to decrease markedly in starvation [59, p. 840]).

- They became easily and markedly depressed.

So similar is the reported experience of these men to that of our patients that one wonders what we are left with to call anorexia nervosa when we subtract the symptoms of starvation. So, back to the question I posed in the opening paragraph of this chapter: Once the cloud of effects caused by food restriction clears, when we forcefully return the patient to a well-fed state, what do we see? We see a delusional belief in self as fat that the MSSS subjects emphatically did not report, we see a paranoid belief that others are attempting to make them fat or are thinking them already fat, and we see an irrational denial of the deleterious effects of weight loss on their health and life. *That* is anorexia nervosa.

## Clinical pearls

- Starved human brains become obsessed with thoughts about food.

- Muscle is lost in starvation, including heart muscle.

- Sociability suffers in starvation.

- Starved people are irritable and lose their sense of humor.

- Starved humans may try to drink large quantities of coffee, tea, or caffeinated soda pop.

- Starvation does not mean not eating at all; it means not eating enough.

# 10 Psychopharmacology

By Janiece Desocio[1]

Rarely do we think about food as having pharmacological properties, but in fact, food is an essential source of the chemicals produced by our brains to stabilize moods, moderate anxiety, induce sleep, reduce pain, and regulate appetite. In this chapter, I will explain how important food is to the optimal functioning of the brain and the production of neurotransmitters, which are the targets of the psychotropic medications we prescribe for mood, anxiety, and attention.

The brain is a natural pharmacy. Most of our psychotropic medications have been designed to regulate the naturally occurring chemicals in our brains. According to Stephen Stahl, a well known psychopharmacologist, the therapeutic action of medications often replicates or mimics the actions of the brain itself, when the brain is working optimally and producing its own chemicals [115]. The goal of psychopharmacology is to work in partnership with these naturally occurring chemicals, referred to as neurotransmitters, to return the brain to an optimal state of functioning. There are as many as 200 different neurotransmitters produced by the brain to regulate behavior, thought, emotion, appetite, growth, and numerous body functions. However, the medications we refer to as "psychotropic" act primarily on just six of these chemical neuro-

[1]Janiece Desocio PhD, RN, PMHNP-BC. Associate Professor of Clinical Nursing, University of Rochester Psychiatric Nurse Practitioner for Kartini Clinic

transmitters: Serotonin, dopamine, norepinephrine, acetylcholine, and GABA (gamma amino butyric acid) [115].

How do these chemical neurotransmitters work to regulate emotions and behavior? The popularity of "instant messaging" (IM) provides a useful metaphor for the communication processes of the brain, which transmit vast numbers of chemical messages every nanosecond. The brain's version of IM is "chemical messaging," which we can refer to as "CM." The cells or "neurons" of the brain communicate with each other through exchange of these chemicals. There are billions of neurons in our brains, each with thousands of connections to other neurons. Our brains are an amazingly dense network of neurons that are continuously communicating by processes of chemical messaging [115].

It is easier to understand how this process works by isolating just two neurons in this complex communication network; a sending neuron and a receiving neuron. Each neuron is set up to both receive and send chemical messages. In order to participate in this CM process, the neuron must have the capacity to produce (synthesize) the chemicals necessary for neurotransmission. The synthesis of these chemicals is under the control of the genetic DNA within the nucleus of each neuron. If the DNA signals the production of serotonin, for example, the neuron synthesizes and stores serotonin in vesicles ("storage units") within the neuron's cell body. When the neuron receives a CM from another neuron, it is "activated" to release its stored serotonin into the "synapse" or the space connecting it with other neurons. The space between neurons is bridged by the release and uptake of chemical neurotransmitters. The receiving neurons have receptors designed for uptake of CMs released by sending neurons. The chemical neurotransmitter and receptor fit together like a key in a lock; if the key fits, it opens or "activates" the receptor on the receiving neuron, and thus the communication chain continues by activation of the receiving neuron, which triggers chemical neurotransmission to subsequent neurons in the communication pathway.

There is one more neuronal process that is important to understand because it is central to how many psychotropic medications work in regulating CM within the brain. This process quite simply represents the brain's efficient use of precious resources through "recycling." Alongside the neuronal vesicles that store the chemical neurotransmitters, each neuron has a recycling unit or "reuptake pump" whose purpose is to retrieve any unused chemical from the synaptic space and pump it back into the storage unit of the sending neuron where it can be saved for future use.

For some individuals, abnormalities in particular genes and chromosomes alter the production, transmission, and/or reuptake of these vital chemicals needed for the brain's CM system. These individuals may be predisposed to problems with anxiety, depression, unstable moods, and other psychiatric disorders. Psychotropic medications are chemical compounds with designed capabilities to bind to neuronal receptors and regulate the chemical messaging system toward more optimal functioning. Serotonin, dopamine, and norepinephrine are among the chemical neurotransmitters linked to eating disorders, as well as many other mental disorders such as depression, anxiety, and obsessive compulsive disorder [34]. The fundamental problem arises from the genetic DNA within the nucleus of each neuron, and the genetic code that signals the neuron's production and expression of chemical neurotransmitters. Genetic studies of families with one or more members affected by eating disorders are attempting to isolate parts of the human genome that play a role in eating disorders. Currently, research has isolated a serotonin receptor gene that is believed to play a role in anorexia nervosa [63], and other studies are beginning to explain the role of dopamine in this disorder [29] [123].

With this basic understanding of the anatomy and physiology of the brain's chemical messaging system, we can now get to the interesting part about the pharmacological properties of food. The essential amino acids in the food we eat are the "precursors" or the basic building blocks used by neurons to synthesize the chemical neurotransmitters, including serotonin and dopamine. Neurons simply cannot produce the chemical neurotransmitters without an adequate supply of essential amino acids such as tryptophan and tyrosine, which are extracted from food. Thus, in states of starvation, the brain's stores of chemical neurotransmitters become depleted and there is not enough ingestion of essential amino acids to allow the brain to replenish its dwindling supply. The CM process begins to slow down and misfire and the neuronal communication networks responsible for regulating behavior, mood, anxiety, attention, and other vital functions begin to fail.

In a state of malnutrition, the failing CM process of the brain can result in dramatic changes in behavior and personality. The behaviors and symptoms that result from a malnourished brain can mimic an array of different mental disorders, including depression, anxiety disorders, and attention deficit disorders. It is not unusual, for example, for symptoms of inattention, poor concentration, depression, irritability, obsessive anxiety and compulsive rituals to increase as weight loss progresses in anorexia nervosa—or in any condition that results in extreme weight loss. If the source of these personality changes is not recognized as the misfiring of a malnourished brain, the individual could inadvertently be given any number of psychiatric diagnoses instead of recognizing that what they have may be a constellation of symptoms which are reversible with weight restoration.

Thus, we return to the basic tenet of this book, "Give food a chance," and emphasize the importance of re-feeding the starved brain so it can replenish its stores of natural brain chemicals before deciding if other mental disorders are present. To repeat: Experience has taught us that children and adolescents with starved brains can look like they have attention deficit disorder, mood disorders, anxiety disorders and even psychotic disorders. Sometimes after re-feeding, we find that the child or adolescent does indeed have both an eating disorder and an anxiety disorder or mood disorder. This is not unusual because we know these disorders share genetic predispositions to serotonin dysregulation and tend to cluster together in genetic families. At other times, symptoms that initially looked like anxiety, depression, psychosis or ADD go away when the child has been restored to nutritional health. So, we have learned to be cautious in diagnosing and treating psychiatric symptoms until we sort out the effects of malnutrition.

Now, back to our discussion of eating disorders, genetics, and psychopharmacology! If eating disorders result from a genetically programmed abnormality in serotonin and other neurotransmitters, shouldn't we use psychopharmacology to re-regulate these chemicals in the brain in order to prevent the onset of restricting symptoms that contribute to a malnourished brain in anorexia nervosa? The answer is yes, BUT there must be enough essential amino acid available from food BEFORE many psychotropic medications can act on the dysregulated CM system. The SSRI antidepressants, for example, are often used to treat anxiety and depression. We believe an individual must be at least 90% of his or her healthy weight before these medications can work effectively [58]. The reason is based on the mechanism of action of the SSRI antidepressants. The acronym SSRI stands for Selective Serotonin Reuptake Inhibitor. Thus, one of the actions, and possibly the primary action of the SSRIs (Prozac, Zoloft, Paxil, Celexa, and Lexapro) is to inhibit or block the neuron's reuptake pump (the recycling pump) so that serotonin remains freely circulating in the synapse for a longer time, allowing more of the receptor sites on receiving neurons to take-up the chemical message. Imagine, for example, if you were a slow eater and someone in your family cleared the table of all food after five minutes. Unless someone could get them to stop and allow food to remain on the table long enough for you to eat enough, you would go hungry. It would not be necessary to make more food, just to allow the food that was already produced to be left on the table long enough for you to access it. The SSRIs do not "make" or "produce" serotonin; their primary job is to slow down recycling, which is downstream from serotonin production.

Slowing down the removal of serotonin from the synapse is one of the jobs of the SSRI. But there's more: Without a sufficient natural supply of the amino acid tryptophan, which is the precursor for serotonin production, the SSRI's job of shutting down the recycle pump is just too little too late. When the brain is sufficiently nourished and is producing its own serotonin again (at about 90% weight for health), the actions of the SSRIs begin to take effect and we can expect to see an improvement in mood and a decrease in anxiety, but probably not until then. There is research evidence that the SSRI antidepressants can extend periods of remission in weight restored individuals with anorexia nervosa, and can decrease binge and purge symptoms in individuals with bulimia nervosa and binge eating disorder [58]. In each of these conditions, the SSRI is effective when the individual weighs at least his or her expected weight for health (or sometimes more, as in the case of binge eating disorder). This makes sense once we understand how the SSRIs work and the more critical role of food and nutrition in supplying the essential amino acids for the brain's production of serotonin before the SSRI can play its part in the CM process.

What other psychotropic medications besides the SSRI's are used in treating anorexia nervosa, and how do they act on the brain CM system? A relatively new class of psychotropic medications, referred to as atypical antipsychotics or second-generation antipsychotics (SGAs) have been found to play a helpful role in the treatment of anorexia nervosa [11] [28]. Eating disorder research has been conducted with several of these medications, including olanzapine, risperidone, and quetiapine [77].

A novel antipsychotic, aripiprazole (Abilify) is just coming on the scene in eating disorder research and literature. While these medications are similar in action, they are also different from each other in both positive effects and undesirable side effects. They are similar in their role of regulating a balance between the activating neurotransmitters dopamine and norepinephrine, and the calming neurotransmitter serotonin.

The limibic area of the brain and structures within the limbic system are recognized as having a central role in regulating anxiety. The feeling of anxiety is incited within the amygdala (a structure of the limbic system) when information from our sensory organs (e.g. our eyes, ears, nose, and skin) signal danger. Anxiety is controlled by the action of our "thinking" brains; primarily the prefrontal cortex, which conducts a thoughtful (yet unbelievably swift) analysis of the source of the danger and communicates to the limbic system to either "calm down" or "get ready to fight or flee." Thus, our brain's "anxiety management system" involves a communication network connecting the limbic system, which lies deep in the center of the brain, with the prefrontal cortex located in the frontal lobe of the brain. The limbic system is richly supplied with neuronal circuits that produce dopamine, norepinephrine, and serotonin, and extend their neuronal branches up to the prefrontal cortex to assure a good connection with the "executive functions" of the "thinking" brain. These top-down connections allow our brains to put on the anxiety brakes when an over-stimulated limbic system is acting like an out-of-control bus approaching a steep decline.

If the dopamine communication network misfires, it can result in a variety of very frightening symptoms. Delusions and hallucinations result from dysregulation of dopamine in the limbic networks of the brain. We see the effects of this in anorexia nervosa, when delusions take the form of distorted thoughts about body size and shape. These distorted thoughts can take on frightening proportions, such as believing the body is insidiously depositing large globules of fat with each mouthful of food, or believing the air and environment are contaminated by evil trans-fats that can be absorbed through the skin (more than one very young child has reported having this particular fear.) Some of our patients with severe anorexia nervosa report auditory hallucinations; hearing "a voice" that forbids them to eat and punishes them with incessant accusations of weakness or failure when they eat even miniscule amounts of food. We believe these symptoms arise from a dysregulated dopamine system in the brain's limbic structures and a failure of the top-down anxiety braking mechanism to rationally modulate anxiety. Interestingly, as the brain becomes more and more malnourished, these symptoms tend to intensify. We have observed this in patients with anorexia nervosa, and also in patients with food phobia. The SGAs are especially designed to regulate the production of dopamine in the limbic centers of the brain, while also balancing serotonin so that the end result is a decrease in delusions and hallucinations, a decrease in anxiety, and a stabilization and improvement in mood. We have found olanzapine and its rapidly dissolving form, to be particularly helpful in achieving these positive effects, even in states of starvation. Relatively small doses of olanzapine (much lower than prescribed for psychotic disorders or bipolar disorder, for example) can be very helpful in reducing the disordered thoughts and alleviating the high anxiety of our patients with anorexia nervosa and food phobia. While we do not fully understand the interaction of food and the restoration of brain health on the effects of the SGA medications, experience has taught us that, for most of our patients, the restoration of a healthy body weight is a marker for when we can begin slowly tapering and discontinuing these SGA medications. For many of our patients with anorexia nervosa, this occurs within the first six to nine months of treatment—for our patients with food phobia, this often occurs much sooner.

As pediatric practitioners we are conservative, cautious prescribers. It is critical to do no harm. We do not hesitate to use medication when we feel it is indicated in order for a child to make progress and be rescued from malnutrition, but we use all medications judiciously and with a plan for discontinuation in order to acquire the greatest potential benefit with the least potential cost in side effects. Recent literature has heightened our awareness of the potential long term effects of the SGAs on metabolism and weight gain, especially when prescribed to children [17]. And although we have not seen these reported effects in our patients, a risk versus benefit analysis is always important in discussing medications with parents. Keep in mind that with severely ill patients with anorexia or food phobia, where the disease is itself life threatening, the use of an SGA can be a life saving measure and can allow the individual sufficient relief from overwhelming anxiety and delusional thoughts to begin accepting nutrition and participating in a treatment process that will return them to health.

Our parents and patients teach us many things, and among our most important lessons has been that the prescription of psychotropic medications must be done in partnership with parents. Parents play a critical role in the safe and appropriate use of psychotropic medications with children and adolescents. Giving medications that alter the brain's chemical messaging system is serious business, and not at all like taking Tylenol once in a while for a headache! We believe the responsibility for safe administration of psychotropic medications should never be turned over to a child or adolescent, even though we can expect protests from them—and sometimes from their parents—that they are old enough to take responsibility for their own medications. To be effective, these medications must be taken at prescribed intervals so that a smooth, steady concentration of medication is available in the brain at all times. If doses are missed or taken at widely varying times, the levels of brain chemicals can dip in response, and cause erratic changes in moods and anxiety. Parents are generally more self-regulated in their daily routines than adolescents who may stay up late and sleep in on weekends—or just forget to take a dose of medication here and there. Thus, parents must assume this important responsibility for assuring that psychotropic medications are taken on time and prescriptions are refilled in a timely manner.

But experience has taught us a few more reasons to always have parents administer medication. One is that anorexia nervosa is a disorder that involves delusional fears and beliefs about fat, shape and weight and knowing that "the medication" will help suppress these thoughts is scary for a patient who believes that only their constant vigilance stands between them and becoming (even more) fat. As one patient put it "Zyprexa takes away 'my edge' and I need that 'edge' not to eat." Older children may also read online that weight gain can be a side effect, although, again it is a side effect that we do not see with our low dose, limited duration of treatment and carefully monitored meal plan. Thus they are reluctant to take the medication and will "forget it," "cheek it," or spit it out.

Additionally we know that people of all ages are compliant with medication only about 50% of the time [45]. Therefore, it is essential that parents become our partners so that brain medications are used in the safest and most effective manner.

When we start a patient on a psychotropic medication, we begin with a low dose and slowly increase the dose over time so that the neurons and receptors in the brain have a chance to gradually accommodate and utilize the medication optimally. An abrupt introduction of a large dose of a psychotropic medication is more likely to cause side effects and increase the patient's resistance to taking medications. Thus our motto for psychotropic medication is "start low and go slow." An abrupt discontinuation can likewise be problematic in producing very uncomfortable discontinuation effects from the sudden absence of chemicals the brain and body have come to rely on for neurotransmission. When it is time to consider discontinuing these medications, the prescriber should create a tapering plan that helps the patient adjust to the slow removal of the medication so that a relapse of eating disorder symptoms (or other disorders) can be avoided whenever possible. Parents help us do a more effective job of managing our patients' response to medications; parents reports and their participation in medication management appointments help us know when and how to adjust medication doses, or when to discontinue a particular medication and try something else.

## Clinical pearls for parents

- Psychotropic medications are selected for their ability to regulate naturally occurring chemicals that are necessary for the optimal functioning of the chemical messaging system (neurotransmission) within the brain.

- Food is medicine! The essential amino acids in the food we eat supply the building blocks for production of the chemical messengers of the brain, e.g. serotonin, dopamine, and norepinephrine.

- The SSRI antidepressants act downstream from serotonin production and cannot be optimally effective until the brain is adequately nourished and the individual is returned to at least approximately 90% of his/her weight for health.

- The second generation antipsychotic medications, such as olanzapine, have research evidence of effectiveness in malnourished states of anorexia nervosa, and can be life saving measures when used judiciously during treatment and restoration of health.

- All psychotropic medications should be administered by parents under the supervision of a psychiatric or medical prescriber. These medications should not be discontinued abruptly to avoid discontinuation side effects, and they should be regularly monitored during appointments with prescribers and through routine laboratory tests.

- Parents are partners in decisions about using psychotropic medications for children and adolescents with eating disorders. The better informed parents are, the greater the potential for achieving positive effects and avoiding undesirable side effects. Always feel free to ask questions and learn as much as possible about your child's psychotropic medications!

## Clinical pearls for prescribers

- Close follow-up is the most important and often the most overlooked responsibility we have. A child's response to psychotropic medication should be monitored carefully in accordance with guidelines of the American Academy of Child and Adolescent Psychiatry.

- Do not let children and teens be in charge of these medications. Ask the parents *every time* when they give the medications and how. Parents need to know you mean business about parental supervision, and why. It is better for a child to have no medication than one that is poorly supervised and erratically taken.

- If you are not comfortable or experienced with the use of psychotropic medications, such as the neuroleptics or antipsychotics, just say no when asked to prescribe.

- Always be aware of the most severe side effects of any medication you prescribe, discuss them with the parents and let them help you be vigilant.

- When new or unexpected symptoms come to your attention, always suspect the medication, or medication interactions. Ask about medications the patient may be using but which you did not prescribe.

- Avoid the use of sleep medication, antacids, laxatives, pain medication, and benzodiazepines for anxiety in children with eating disorders.

- An online database or consultation with a pharmacist can prove to be a big help. Encourage parents to fill all their child's prescriptions at the same pharmacy so that any drug interactions among prescription drugs will be immediately flagged on the pharmacy database.

- Herbs and herbals such as ginseng, St. John's Wort, and many, many others have as many potential interactions as physician-prescribed medications do and yet people are much more cavalier about using them. An online database such as Epocrates can prove a big help with this.

# 11 What is the role of family?

Our treatment philosophy at the Kartini Clinic can be summarized as follows:

- Anorexia nervosa is a brain disorder.

- Parents did not cause it.

- Children do not choose to have it.

- Parental unity with the team is critical.

- Doctors and parents are in charge.

- Weight restoration is the cornerstone of treatment. *If you do not achieve this, you will achieve nothing.*

- All families participate in family therapy/education.

- All meal preparation and all shopping will be done by parents alone.

- Family dinners will become a part of every meal plan.

- Parents are responsible for recording and bringing all food journals to every appointment. We tell them: "If you do not bring your food journal, you will not be seen."

- All patients, unless specifically cleared by the team, do group therapy.

- We will not continue to treat a patient whose parents refuse the best medical advice of the physicians about intensity of treatment (i.e. hospitalization if needed, residential placement referral if needed, day treatment if needed, medication if indicated).

The cornerstone of our treatment philosophy is our belief that parents and families are not the problem, but an essential part of the solution. This is so true that I literally have no idea how to treat a child who has no family. Sadly, I'm not even sure it can be done. When I founded the Kartini Clinic and our family-based mode of treatment there was no widely available "Maudsley Approach" to the treatment of pediatric eating disorders. Through the work of Laura Collins (*Eating with Your Anorexic*) I became aware of a large number of parents who have dedicated themselves and their family to re-feeding their own eating disordered child. In some cases it is because they cannot find appropriate family-oriented treatment, in others because they cannot afford it, and others simply prefer it. When it works, I say "hats off!" Who am I to criticize success? We do not practice the "Maudsley Method" at the Kartini Clinic and I will not go into any reservations I have about it. If you are a "Maudsley parent" and it is working for your child, I am thrilled. But you are probably not reading this book if that is the case, because you do not need it. If Maudsley has not worked for you, or it worked initially but remission has not been complete or perhaps not lasting or perhaps bingeing or excessive weight gain has become an issue and you wonder why, the approach we have to offer may be of some use.

It has become fashionable to say that adequate treatment of eating-disordered patients requires a multidisciplinary team and approach. Having tried other approaches in the past, I can assert that this is more than just the fashionable thing to say—it is the truth. It takes a team, and the approach must be not only multidisciplinary but holistic. The term *multidisciplinary* places emphasis on the providers or types of providers; the term *holistic* places the emphasis on the patients. Viewing the patient, the child, as a whole is what it means to have an holistic approach.

It has likewise become fashionable to say that a contemporary approach to the treatment of eating disorders needs to be a *biopsychosocial* approach. I might amend this to a BIOpsychosocial approach, since, in the end, all approaches need to be rooted in our biology. Having said that, however, we are not robots: We are complex beings with feelings, beliefs, concerns, fears, and hopes, and to act as if we are not is to perpetuate the great weaknesses of Western medicine. For this reason, although our approach to the treatment of childhood eating disorders at the Kartini Clinic is strongly based in medical treatment, we also pull in "heart and mind" and "mind and body" specialists to make up our treatment teams.

One common form of "treatment team" consisting of, for example, a generalist physician, a therapist, and a nutritionist is not, in our view, an adequate team at all. For one thing such a "team" will not be under one roof. A "team" made up of providers from different clinics simply does not have enough hours in the day for all members to communicate as much and as often as they need to about a given eating-disordered patient. Complex issues requiring complex planning, such as the return to college, demand a high level of cooperative treatment. Additionally, one therapist or one nutritionist or physician is often forced to work with a different constellation of the other two providers for each different patient, which adds to the complexity of communication and the possibilities of treatment approach splitting. This treatment team triad (doctor, therapist, nutritionist), often resorted to for lack of a nearby specialized clinic, is, in our experience, so unsuccessful we have come to call it "the deadly triad" when used for initial assessment. Our clinic is filled with patients who have failed with this approach, and we consider it fully inadequate to care for children or adolescents with anorexia nervosa. Although I am aware that this belief on our part will not be a popular one, there is no way to escape our observation over the years that, in the case of pediatric anorexia nervosa, the triad of providers just mentioned often merely become witnesses to the child's gradual decline. Whether or not "Maudsley" teams will be any different remains to be seen. Reports to date involve such small numbers of patients it is hard to be sure.

What of patients who live in areas far removed from specialist care? This is no different from the situation for those pediatric patients who need heart surgery or cancer therapy. If they must travel to get care, it is definitely a hardship, but one that the family must be prepared to meet and the insurance company to sanction.

When I was a general pediatrician seeing patients with eating disorders, I learned a lot. I learned that these patients could be scheduled for thirty minutes and need ninety. I learned that they not uncommonly needed hospitalization, requiring a lengthy discussion with their parents, just about the same time as I would be called to the delivery room. I learned that my partners were not happy to have to deal with the "psychosocial" issues that came up on the weekends with their families when they were in the hospital'. I learned that it was not possible to get community psychotherapists to make rounds on eating-disorder patients on the weekends or after hours in the hospital, or usually to see them at all in that setting. I learned that when I called the treating mental health professional, unlike calling another physician, they could not be interrupted during session and often would not return calls until the end of the day or the following one. I learned that general pediatric office nurses would weigh these patients in their clothes, or tell them enthusiastically how they had gained weight, or lecture them about "getting over it," or advise them to "just eat." I learned that eating-disorder patients would water-load in the clinic bathrooms, or vomit there, or run up and down the stairs when nervous, or wear weights in their clothes. In other words, they did not do well in the setting of a general practice with busy nurses and doctors who were trying to care for crying children needing urgent care. But most of all I learned that, at the end of the day, there was no one under the same roof to talk to me about our very special patients when I was discouraged, puzzled, or alarmed. It just didn't work.

It takes a team.

And it takes a family [92].

At the Kartini Clinic, over the years, we have made just about all mistakes. One thing we have learned never to do, no matter how tempted we are to care for a "high-profile" patient, is to accept care of a child whose parents will not be involved. It just doesn't work.

Without a supportive adult caretaker, the prognosis for an eating-disordered child or young adult is grim. I discuss the special situation for young adults at greater length in the chapters on the Day Treatment Unit (also called "Intensive Outpatient" in some institutions or "Partial Hospital" in others), but for now let me say that *parental unity with the team* has proven to be the critical, the essential, ingredient in successful treatment: *Parents and doctors in coalition, against the disease, on behalf of the child.* Nothing else works as well, in our experience.

Over the years we have also earned to avoid what can only be called "enabling" of the eating disorder. This occurs when the patient is allowed (by the doctor) to stay at a suboptimal weight because parents are unable to supervise meals adequately or cannot be convinced to keep a food journal or cannot bear their child's distress at weight gain. It occurs when families refuse family therapy participation because they insist that their child is "the one with the problem," or when families demand outpatient treatment (or doctors propose it) when the child is too medically compromised to benefit from it. Over the years we have watched individual therapists, physicians and nutritionists continue to see terribly compromised patients in an outpatient setting in the belief that "some treatment is better than none," with the result that the child is enabled to remain in a limbo of partial weight restoration. This situation, although not good for adults either, is particularly grave for children, who have a finite window of opportunity to achieve normal growth and brain development and to lay down bone mass. It is essential that parents find providers who have the courage of their convictions and will act in their child's best interest. You need a doctor who will give it to you straight, not be afraid to tell you what you may not want to hear. Parents are a child's best advocates. Doctors: Tell parents what they need to know and what they will have to do and then be there for them when things get difficult.

## 11.1   Unity within the team

Anorexia nervosa is a tough illness to treat. Just ask parents who have tried it alone. We have found that 1) parents and doctors must take charge, and 2) the treatment needs to proceed holistically. To say that our medical doctors are in charge (an adolescent medicine physician and pediatrician in the case of the Kartini Clinic) is not to minimize the role of our mental health professionals, but rather to emphasize, for all concerned, the medical (brain disorder) nature of this eating disorder. For all the reasons outlined in Chapter 1 about former treatment paradigms, we try to *de-stigmatize* this disorder by shifting our focus away from the traditional mental health approach even though all our patients are co-managed by our own team of mental health professionals as described in the next few chapters.

At the same time that our patients are sufferers of anorexia nervosa they are normal children as well. They do things typical of children with eating disorders, and they do things typical of normal children. One behavior that overlaps both realms is what mental health professionals refer to, somewhat politically incorrectly, as "splitting," which every parent will recognize.

To shake off the control and scrutiny of the doctors, the patient will often first try to split one parent from the other, going for the "softer one" in an effort to avoid cooperating with weight gain. Unless the parents can achieve a tight, unified working relationship on behalf of their child (whether happily married, never married, or acrimoniously divorced), treatment stands no chance of working.

If splitting the parents does not work, the child may try to split the parents from their treatment team: "I don't like that doctor!" "Treatment will interfere with my schooling." "She just wants me to be fat like her!" "I'm not like the other kids in the program!" "I'll eat, I swear, just let me go home and do this on my own with you," and so on.

As a last resort, a scared and conflicted child or teen may try to split the team members from one another: "But Dr. X said I could run track," "But my therapist said I don't have to!" and so on. Being aware of this common behavior is our only defense against it. Talking about it ahead of time with parents is the only chance we have of aborting it. Often when it is explained to parents, such behavior is familiar to them from normal childhood behaviors, all kids try at home. *Remember: Parents and team in coalition against the disease, on behalf of the child.*

## Clinical pearls

- Anorexia nervosa is a brain disorder: Neither parent nor child is to blame.

- Parental unity with the team is essential.

- Doctors and parents are in charge.

- Weight restoration is the cornerstone of treatment.

- Family meals are non-negotiable.

- Parents are in charge of all food preparation and oversight.

- All families participate in family therapy.

- The food journal is an anxiety-reduction tool for the kids.

- Doctors monitor and balance caloric intake and weight.

# 12 What should I expect when my child is first evaluated?

From a parent's point of view the first encounter with a specialist eating disorder doctor can be critical. Almost certainly parents are very stressed. They may be uncertain that their child actually has an eating disorder, or if so, how severe it is. They may be afraid to find out how ill their child has become and feel intensely guilty when they do. They may not like doctors. They may be suspicious of therapists. In our country there are also stresses caused by the financial implications of medical care.

What is it like from the doctor's point of view? What should be covered in an ideal "eating disorder" consult? Below I have described our process in detail, which you may want to use to either prompt your physician team or to compare what experience you may have had. It is written as if to another doctor who is learning how to do such an interview.

The Kartini Clinic is a private clinic, entirely dependent on reimbursement within the insurance and private-payment world of the United States and has no outside funding. We must be state of the art, efficient, and always medically correct. I have sat in on admirable academic consults that take half a day or even all day, but such an approach is not possible in a private setting, except for the very wealthy. Our challenge is to get access to the information needed to make an initial diagnosis and assessment of medical stability, to meet the child and *both* parents (whenever possible), to introduce them to our philosophy of treatment, and occasionally to obtain informed consent if they are to be asked to participate in research efforts. Parents must have an opportunity to talk about their concerns and tell us about what they and their child have been through. The child's anxieties about what the doctor is about to "do to them" must be allayed. Working at top speed with an experienced team this process takes about two hours.

## 12.1   Preconsult

Before the doctors ever see a patient, the parents have had an interview with our intake coordinator, who tells them a little about our approach to treatment. Where possible we want parents to understand as much as they can about us before we even meet them, to decrease their sense of surprise, panic, or powerlessness. Our team's mission is to empower them to help us—their team—care for their child. To this end they (and their referring doctor) are referred to our website www.kartiniclinic.com. And God bless the internet! They can read every word I have written in my blog, "meet" our team members, click on related websites, and view the DVD made by the Kartini Foundation (called *Spotting the Tiger*) before they ever see us. They are sent a thick packet of forms to fill out, detailing their child's medical and growth history as well as their own family history. With a heritability of 70%, the family history is very important in anorexia nervosa and will be gone over in detail. Our doctors and therapists always read this documentation ahead of the consultation, which we have asked the parents to fill out as meticulously as possible. I wonder, have you ever been to a doctor's office and asked to fill out a lot of medical information which the doctor does not even look at? I personally have been disappointed and angered by waiting months to see a specialist who did not even bother to read my history, review my labs or X-rays, or even be sure they were available. A consulting specialist should know a lot about the patient before they ever touch them.

## 12.2   Arrival and vitals

When the family arrives at Kartini Clinic, they sign release-of-information forms so that we may confer with other providers who have cared for or are caring for this child. Patients 18 years old or older are asked to sign a release so that we can share information with their parents. Without this we cannot treat young adult patients with our family-based approach and will not do so unless there are extenuating circumstances (such as an abusive parent). This sharing of information does not include a patient's sexual history.

The patient is then taken back to be weighed in a gown, after a void (leaving a urine sample), with their back to the scale. At this initial visit the doctor may choose to discuss their weight, mostly to get an emotional response during the interview and to explore the child's own feelings about their size, but after this initial consult their weight will not be revealed to them again. Over the years, we have discovered that to talk about weight numbers is to inevitably focus the entire discussion on those numbers.

We are a pediatric clinic, so our staff bends over backward to make sure even very young children are comfortable with vitals being taken. Tympanic temperature (using an ear thermometer) and resting heart rate are taken. If the heart rate is 50 BPM or below, the doctor is notified and an EKG is done. Then orthostatic pulse and blood pressure measurements are taken: Five minutes of lying down followed by two and a half of standing. We are not interested in the first flash of "dizziness" many people experience immediately upon suddenly standing up, but rather in determining whether or not the cardiovascular system has been compromised by semi-starvation. Can the heart accommodate to the upright position where it has to work harder to "pump uphill?" Patients over the age of about 11 fill out a BDI (Beck Depression Inventory), a short self-report questionnaire whose score can help assess any depression but which we largely use to help focus the doctor's general questions. The doctor reviews the BDI for his or her own purposes, although we do not use it to make a definitive diagnosis of depression. My experience has been that eating-disordered patients show "false positives" on three parameters on the BDI: "Past failure," "self-dislike," and "self-criticalness" even when depression is not present. Any definitive diagnosis of depression is made later by our psychiatric provider.

While the patient's vitals are being taken, the doctor and the family therapist may review the records forwarded to us (at our request) from the referring physician(s) or therapist(s). We sometimes have difficulty getting written records from mental health providers, even with the patient's express permission, but we always try. We also review the family questionnaire, included in Appendix B.

## 12.3 Physical exam

At this point the two providers split up: The family therapist interviews the parents and the physician interviews the child. It has been my experience that when the doctor is in the room, parents focus on her/him. We want our family therapist's roll validated right from the start. Conversely, the children often expect a mental health interview, having been told they "need help from a therapist." I am quick to point out that, although I am a doctor, I am a pediatrician (and adolescent medicine doctor), not a psychiatrist. They often visibly relax. Then I say, "I am going to do two things with your help, and I will tell you what I am going to do before I do it. I will do your complete exam, but it will not involve blood drawing, needles, or a pelvic exam. Then I am going to ask you a lot of questions and let you ask me anything you want. Okay?" Naturally I gear the tone and vocabulary to the patient's age, as all pediatricians do. Then I say, "In this clinic we are mostly interested in the brain." I have therefore set the stage for de-stigmatizing any eating problems they may turn out to have and make it clear that whatever they tell me, I will not blame them for it. I assure them that they are not to blame for their difficulties throughout the entire exam.

The exam is indeed focused on the brain. We do as thorough a neurological exam as we can, including testing for sense of smell with a small vial of eucalyptus oil. We then look for lanugo, Russell's Sign (small scars or calluses over the knuckles of the dominant hand from inducing vomiting with a finger), muscle wasting, signs of self-mutilation, capillary fill, signs of dehydration, regression of the secondary sexual characteristics (breast tissue wasting) stretch marks from weight fluctuations, protrusion of the spinal bones with bruising (from over-exercising on the floor), enlargement of the lymph nodes or salivary glands, and dental enamel erosion, as well as the usual physical exam findings. When that is over, I offer them a thick blanket and say, "You look cold to me," which they almost always validate. Then I leave while they get dressed and on my return begin the actual interview.

# 12.4   REDS Interview

An eating-disorder interview could stretch over hours, but we do not have hours. For this reason we use the REDS (Rating of Eating Disorder Severity) semi-structured interview. It allows the practitioner to direct the conversation so that he or she covers all the ground needed to make a (provisional) diagnosis and a decision about treatment.

## The REDS-Child (rating of eating disorder severity) semi-structured interview

I begin the REDS-C questions by asking things not overtly related to eating disorders. If, at this point, you can make the patient laugh, you are home free. If not, be sure your tone is one of compassion and empathy throughout. Have a box of tissues handy. Although some, mostly older, patients are too guarded to give honest answers, most kids are scared by their eating problems on some level and are anxious (sometimes proud!) to tell their story. I ask about their year in school. I ask about their grades—not because I care but because they usually do. Patients with anorexia nervosa are almost always high achievers. For those patients whose grades are not good (often those struggling with impulsive behaviors), make it a subject of rueful empathy: "I got a D in calculus once myself. Ouch."

If you are interviewing a patient with an eating problem of any kind, please take a minute history, not just a general one, of what the patient eats, but try to bury your food questions within a question such as "Give me a day in the life of Susie..." Carefully write down what time they say they get up and what classes they take so that they are not startled when you write down what they eat. Salt your interview with some "red herring questions" to put them at their ease and so they do not get the impression that you are interested only in their eating-disorder-related symptoms and not in their life or concerns. Never neglect to ask about their friends and boyfriends/girlfriends. When you ask about sex, let them know that this information will not be shared with their parents unless you discover they have been hurt or threatened and that even then, you will reveal this to parents with their participation, if they prefer. Don't ask if they are "sexually active" (what does *that* mean?) Ask if they have "ever had sex." If they say no, ask if they "have ever come close." If they say no, ask if that means they have had oral sex but not vaginal sex (common these days), although you are well advised to use some sensitivity to the child's age. If they say yes, remember this for future reference to let the therapists know, so the team can understand what this particular young person's life is really like, but don't write it anywhere where the information may not be protected.

When talking about purging (vomiting) try to use the passive voice. Don't say, "Are you doing this?" But rather, "Is this happening to you?" Bingeing is very humiliating. Let them know that in an eating-disorder clinic bingeing and purging are not things to be embarrassed about, because many people suffer from them. Instead frame it that bingeing and purging in an eating-disorder clinic is like coughing in a pulmonary clinic: Just a common symptom. And mean it.

Once I am satisfied with the REDS interview, I thank them for doing such a great job answering questions. Then I tell them that I will now go meet their parents and that once I have, I will come and get them so we can all discuss next steps together.

## 12.5    Parental consult

By this time the family therapist is finished with the parents. If not, I wait. If I already know, based on the vitals, that this patient requires hospitalization, I take this time to notify the ward of a probable admission. I may even write orders and fetch a parent handbook for the parents. Once the family therapist can step out of the room for a few minutes, we briefly and succinctly compare notes. It takes two minutes. We return to the family, and I introduce myself to the parents, who have been with the therapist until now. I usually say something such as, "What a wonderful son/daughter  you have. He/she did a good job answering my questions."  Just make sure that whatever you say is sincere. Parents will often choke up at this, because they are likely to have been through a lot by this time.

The next words out of my mouth will be to explain that although I think their child has an eating disorder (assuming I do), *it is not their fault.* Now both parents tear up, even otherwise stoic fathers. It never ceases to amaze me how much blame parents have either been assigned or have self-assigned before I meet them. This up-front "no blame" approach is never more important than when the parents do not get along, because they may feel compelled to blame each other.

# 12.6   Hospitalization

If I think the child needs hospitalization, I come right to the point. Because we are a tertiary care (specialized children's hospital setting) pediatric eating-disorder center for the Pacific Northwest, more than half of first-time patients are ill enough to require hospitalization at the first visit. Parents are often shocked. I now explain the ramifications of bradycardia (low heart rate), extreme inanition (wasting), orthostasis (extreme change in pulse and/or blood pressure with standing), syncope (fainting), or whatever my chief concern is. I explain that, although this may be a shock to them, the inpatient *induction of re-feeding* is the ideal. I tell them I know what they have been through and that it is our belief that re-feeding in a *very ill* child can't be done safely at home both because the child is almost certain to continue to refuse and because of the potential for re-feeding syndrome [101] [39]. I tell them I know they have done everything they could. At this point they invariably ask if their child knows about the hospitalization and I say no. In the Kartini Clinic, I explain, we believe that in the family the parents are in charge; we do not confer with our patients and exclude the family, as is common in mental health clinics. We will explain to the child the need for hospitalization with the parents present. The exception to this might be with the young adult patient where I sometimes begin to introduce the idea before I meet with the parents.

At this point parents almost invariably say something like "She will be devastated," often adding, "She has a trip to Disneyland with her class/the lead in the school play/her SAT test/a tennis tournament/a swim meet /[fill in the blank]." We point out that this would be the case if my news were that she had a brain tumor: A regrettable loss of important activities, but necessary nonetheless. I then tell them: "Many of our patients, when told they need hospitalization, are not shocked and devastated, they are relieved." We see time and again that patients know they are in more trouble than they are letting on and that they are, in fact, relieved to have a doctor announce that from now on they will be kept safe.

Occasionally, but rarely, we have a patient who announces that they will not go in the hospital. I explain that hospitalization is a medical decision, made with their parents' consent, on their behalf, and that it is not negotiable. It is a matter of safety. I do not mention weight; I focus on the heart. And I focus on it loud and clear. If they still refuse angrily, saying, "I'll run away," we call security and have a visible escort to the hospital. It sends a message, and they are just children. Only once or twice have we had to place a two-physician hold and then only with an adult patient. If they say, "I will kill myself if you put me in the hospital," we explain to the parents and child that we can keep only those eating-disordered patients on the pediatric/adolescent medical floor who are safe and behaviorally contained. Other patients will have to go on the locked psychiatric ward and be cared for by other providers. We are not above a security escort to the emergency room for a psychiatric safety evaluation when needed. Our overwhelming experience, however, is that if the doctor and parents present hospitalization as a *safety issue, not a weight issue,* the child will go reluctantly but cooperatively. They are scared.

What do we do when a parent refuses hospitalization for their child? There is not much we can do. If, after explaining our medical concerns to the parents, they still refuse hospitalization, we have to send them back to their family physician and wish them luck with another team. We cannot and should not engage in substandard medical care.

# 12.7 Outpatient follow-up

Because greater than 70% of our first-time patients need inpatient hospitalization, it follows that less than 30% do not. At the time of this writing we almost never agree to follow a patient in the outpatient clinic initially. There is simply too much to learn for both the child and the whole family to effectively re-feed them by seeing them once a week or even a few times a week. If the child does not meet hospitalization criteria, they are usually placed in the Day Treatment Unit (DTU) for re-feeding and teaching and to introduce them to the therapist(s) who will be working with them. I am, of course, aware that there are parents who successfully refeed their own children at home—and more power to them– but specialty clinics like ours are for those in whom this approach has not proven practical.

Admission directly to the Day Treatment Unit (DTU) from home is called a *step-up admission* as opposed to when the child is stepped down from inpatient hospitalization to the DTU, called *step-down admission*. Most treatment facilities that offer day treatment are very familiar with "step-up" versus "step-down" and are aware that "step-up" is much harder to make successful than "step-down." Why? Psychologically, if the patient goes from the hospital to the DTU (where they are home at night and on the weekends), it seems like a vast improvement, whereas if they go from doing as they please at home to the DTU, having never been in the hospital, it seems a little like prison. Since what matters most is attitude, this makes treatment much harder. Additionally, when a patient has been in the "peaceful, friendly, no-negotiation atmosphere" of the inpatient ward, they have had time to accept and adjust to the fact that eating everything placed in front of them is the way it has to be. If it were up to us, any young patient who met criteria for anorexia nervosa—medically stable or not—would first be admitted to the hospital for the induction of re-feeding and then stepped down through the day treatment unit to outpatient as quickly as possible. This would give the greatest opportunity for teaching and achieve the most stable results. In today's insurance climate in the United States such an approach is still simply out of the question.

How treatment is begun and in which setting is the first very important decision made together with parents. The Kartini team makes every attempt to get it right the first time.

## Clinical pearls

- Include the family therapist right from the start.

- Assure the child and the parents that none of this is their fault.

- Explain what your treatment team has to offer, and set the tone of "parents and doctors in charge" from the beginning.

- Discuss the fact that medications may have to be used.

- Always do a complete physical exam, including neurological exam and Tanner (SMR) staging. This is more important than lab tests.

- Starting treatment as an inpatient in the hospital actually helps the patient accept subsequent treatment and makes life easier for the parents.

# 13 My child has to go to the hospital?

A strong inpatient service is essential to the care of young people with anorexia nervosa. Prior to the founding of the Kartini Clinic there was no medical inpatient care for children with eating disorders in the Pacific Northwest. Once the diagnosis of an eating disorder was made and a child needed hospital care, this was done either on an emergent basis by generalist physicians or on locked psychiatric wards. There were no standardized admission criteria, and, despite severe medical complications, these were considered "mental health" admissions, leaving many (if not most) people hugely underinsured for the care. Worse, repeat hospitalization was the norm, with ill children and adolescents being stabilized briefly before being discharged home to further restricting or binge-ing and purging, only to reappear in short order in the emergency room. Such intense half-medical/half-psychiatric hospitalizations were scary and frustrating for the providers, and few were interested in caring for these children. Even today there are institutions who purport to care for eating disordered children and adolescents but who do not offer inpatient medical stabilization. In this chapter I have gone into a great deal of detail, some of which may be confusing to a parent who, after all, is only dealing with their own individual child. But parents motivated to get the best, most up-to-date information and care for their child will probably be glad to have "the whole picture." Some parents even copy the information for their treatment team's use.

As mentioned before, Stanford University's adolescent medicine and psychiatric teams at Lucille Packard Children's Hospital fundamentally changed the situation regarding lack of insurance coverage for northern California with the institution of their standardized criteria for *medical admission*. Children were no longer admitted for "anorexia nervosa," but rather for "bradycardia," "orthostasis," "hypokalemia," etc., not in an attempt to fool the insurance companies, but in an attempt to wrest adequate care from a system that allotted mental health care such a tiny fraction of benefits that no one could be adequately stabilized. Despite the initial frustrating difficulties with the insurance companies discussed earlier, I was able slowly to forge a working relationship with some of them, based on adherence to the strict medical admission criteria and an "open book" policy with their medical directors, which allowed our patients to be stabilized before definitive treatment in a less intensive setting.

## 13.1   When to admit

In 2003 the American Academy of Pediatrics (AAP) [54] formalized and expanded the hospital criteria that the Kartini Clinic, Schneider Children's Hospital, Stanford University, and others had been using, and although no standardized criteria are perfect or unassailable, this has made an organized approach to medical care of children with any wasting disorders possible. Admission criteria are listed below and discussed individually. These are the same AAP Guidelines I discussed earlier as signs of potential eating disorders, but here they are discussed in more detail as hospital admission criteria:

## AAP guidelines

**Anorexia nervosa:**

- Bradycardia: Heart rate <50 beats per minute daytime; <45 beats per minute nighttime.

- Orthostasis: Orthostatic changes in pulse (>20 beats per minute) or blood pressure (>10 mm Hg).

- <75% ideal body weight  , or ongoing weight loss despite intensive management.

- Refusal to eat.

- Body fat <10%.

- Temperature <96° $F$.

- Systolic pressure <90 mmHg.

- Cardiac arrhythymias.

**Bulimia nervosa (or any purging eating disorder):**

- Syncope.

- Serum potassium concentration <3.2 mmol/L.

- Serum chloride concentration <88 mmol/L.

- Esophageal tears.

- Hematemesis (vomiting blood).

- Intractable vomiting.

- Cardiac arrhythmias, including prolonged QTc.

- Hypothermia.

- Suicide risk.

- Failure to respond to outpatient treatment.

Now in detail those criteria which we use at the Kartini Clinic, written for doctors, but meant to be clear for parents:

1. **Heart rate less than or equal to 50 BPM during the day and 45 BPM at night.** If there were only one test available to you in the evaluation of a child, it should be taking a resting heart rate. This is a very important hospitalization criterion. If a child's heart rate on presentation meets criteria, we hospitalize them right away. Is this because we think they will die imminently? No. Very likely the child's cardiovascular system has slowly adapted to this low heart rate, because it is a direct consequence of starvation. We admit them to the hospital because we view this bradycardia as a MARKER for degree of physical compromise related to semi-starvation.

   It is worth noting that the very low heart rates seen with semi-starvation are—in my experience—almost entirely independent of the child's athletic status, *because they always normalize with adequate re-feeding.* Even if some elite adult athletes (some of whom may be eating disordered) have extraordinarily low heart rates, children and teens are not meant to. Once again, we know this because we observe them returning to normal levels with food alone.

The AAP recommends hospitalization if the daytime heart rate is 50 BPM or below OR the nighttime heart rate is less than or equal to 45 BPM [54]. For years we used a lower daytime cutoff (45 BPM). However, our current practice, in line with these recommendations is to admit the child with a heart rate of 50 BPM during office hours. We place them on telemetry (continuous wireless monitoring). This way, we are able to get a clearer picture of how low the heart rate actually goes overnight and in the early morning hours. If the heart rate stays at 45 and above overnight, and this is their only medical instability criterion, we feel we can safely discharge them to re-feeding in the Day Treatment Unit. If not, we know they are well placed on the inpatient ward.

A child seen in the doctor's office during the day is often nervous or angry, sometimes having just drunk a coffee drink, "energy drink," or caffeinated diet soda, and if their heart rate is 50 BPM or less, you know you are seeing the PEAK rate, and not a resting rate at all. It is easy to be fooled into thinking they are less bradycardic than they really are [95]. Unless you specifically ask what they are drinking during the day, they are unlikely to mention it. If the history for caffeinated beverages is negative, ask the parents. I recently asked a 19-year-old new patient whether or not she drank caffeinated beverages. She said no. Her parents told me they were buying Red Bull © for her by the case every week (Red Bull=80 mg of caffeine in 8.2 oz, as compared with 40 mg in 1 oz. of espresso).

A family history of low heart rate has no bearing on the initial evaluation of low heart rate in the face of semi-starvation. However, parents may not accept this. Sometimes we have no choice but to ask for the parents' medical records. Every time we have done this, the parent did turn out to have a lower than average heart rate: 50-55 BPM!

2. **Orthostatic pulse change of greater than or equal to 35 BPM or a drop in systolic blood pressure of 10 mmHg from lying for 5 minutes to standing for 2 1/2 minutes.** You can see immediately that these criteria differ a little from those of the AAP. Based on our own clinical practice, we accept more pulse differential. There is, in fact, some minor variation in numbers when it comes to what pulse and blood pressure changes are acceptable across the country [126]. Neville Golden *et al.* report in their study of 36 adolescent patients in 2003 to have used a blood pressure drop of 20 mmHg as a cut-off and a rise in pulse rate of 20 BPM. At the Kartini Clinic we set the bar higher for pulse changes because, in our clinical experience, we would have to hospitalize too many patients, some of whom we could handle in the Day Treatment Unit. If a strong Day Treatment program (DTU) is not in place at your institution, your treatment team may need to handle this more conservatively and I would recommend strict adherence to the AAP guidelines.

Golden *et al.* noted, as have we, that orthostasis worsens initially with re-feeding and that for most people orthostasis takes about three weeks to resolve. I explain to patients and parents that this is because we "rock the metabolic boat" in patients adjusted to semi-starvation [59, p. 338-339]. Again, we hospitalize such patients for orthostasis not because we believe they will likely suffer sudden death, but because this degree of cardiovascular instability is a MARKER for severity of illness [106]. Remember: *Syncope* (fainting) is one of the most common ways for an eating-disordered child to present to the pediatrician, family practitioner, or cardiologist.

3. **Weight <75% of ideal body weight (IBW) or ongoing weight loss despite intensive management.** Virtually every child we see in a tertiary referral center has "ongoing weight loss despite intensive management," but we do not need to hospitalize all of them because we have a very strong day treatment program (DTU). Where this is not the case, further outpatient treatment would be inappropriate for those children with "ongoing weight loss despite intensive management." Such patients need either inpatient hospitalization or referral to a residential treatment program or DTU.

For primary care providers who see children with weight loss, it has been my experience that much too much time and health is lost during a lengthy "wait and see" trial of re-feeding at home. Unless by using Maudsley or other well organized strategies, the parents are able to achieve steady weight gain at home; they should be referred to a center known to be able to do so.

In using the "weight <75% of IBW" criterion, however, the problem arises in making a determination of "ideal body weight." It is important to realize that there is no need to establish a definitive ideal weight goal at the time of hospitalization, as this may change with time. "Ideal body weight," "minimum weight for health," or "expected body weight" is *always an educated guess on the part of the doctor.* Over time, the body itself will tell us when we are at "ideal" by the restoration of functioning, growth, menses, and so on.

Let me digress for a moment and introduce the concept of "establishing ideal body weight" as it will be essential to understanding this admission criteria (<75% IBW), which is sometimes the only criterion we have.

*Determining ideal body weight* in children who suffer from anorexia nervosa is complex. Pediatric patients cannot be treated like "little adults." An example of this principle is the way medication is dosed in childhood. The right dose of an antibiotic for a newborn is different than the right dose for a two year old or for a 14 year old. And so it is for setting "weight goals" in pediatric eating disorder patients.

Bear with me then, because this is not simple. And not only is it not simple, but it is even more complicated and fraught with "special cases" than the following summary would indicate. Yet, I believe, parents and providers can use it as a general guide.

A true discussion of goal weights cannot be separated from knowledge of a child's developmental stage. Have they gone through puberty? If so, is puberty complete? Has breast development begun (if a girl)? Has she ever had a period?

Children, like adults, will fall along some kind of a bell curve of normal weights: The vast majority will be in the average range with some being in the "obese" range and some being in the "growth-stunted" range where the eating disorder struck at a very young age causing stunting of both height and weight (and probably brain growth). I will address these groups below:

I. **Group One: Children who were a normal or average weight before the onset of their anorexia**

**nervosa.** These children need to be divided further into four sub-categories:

A. Those who have not yet begun puberty.

B. Those who are in early to mid puberty with some breast and pubic hair development (if a girl) or pubic and penile development (if a boy).

C. Those who seem to have full breast and pubic hair development but who may have had only one or a very few periods (if a girl) or who seem to have adult pattern pubic hair, but are not shaving and/or do not have adult pattern underarm hair (if a boy).

D. Those who had completed puberty and had two years of menstruation (if a girl) or who had completed puberty and had been shaving (if a boy) before the onset of their eating disorder.

Group A will have the most uncompleted growth potential. Their "goal weight" is a moving target. First return them to the highest weight they have ever experienced. Then go up. You will be looking for normalization of heart rate, blood pressure, temperature, and soon, resumption of height growth. Do not consider your child "done with gaining weight" until they are done with height growth or until they have had normal periods for two years (if a girl) or are shaving (if a boy).

Group B will also still be growing, though some of their growth will be behind them. Look at their growth chart and see what percentile they were growing along two years before you think the eating disorder started. You want this cushion of two years because research shows that, in retrospect, the eating disorder often started much earlier than anyone knew. Aim now for that weight which will return them to this previous percentile and be aware that they will need to continue to gain more weight as they gain height.

Group C will have some, if reduced, height potential, but still have growing brains! Return them to their previous growth percentile and expect them to need to put on a little more weight if they get taller.

Group D will be kids who were fully grown in height before their eating disorder started (but don't forget that brain growth continues). Return them to their highest pre-eating disorder weight. Unless they were objectively obese, resist the temptation to give in to their pleas to be returned to a weight lower than they weighed before their anorexia nervosa, no matter who in the family or circle of friends "weighs that little and they are ok." Remember also that you cannot alleviate anxiety by allowing your child to keep a "lower-end weight" since there is no weight low enough to appease the eating disorder. It's about health. Period.

II. **Group Two: Children who were obese before the onset of their eating disorder.** These children represent a special case. No one wants to return a child to an obese state. If this was the case for your child please understand that your weight goals will be educated guesses and fraught with more anxiety than normal. A formerly obese child is subjectively afraid of "becoming fat" as all eating disordered children are and objectively afraid of it, too. In these cases we look at the family height and weight pattern, the child's growth pattern as a younger child and begin our climb up towards a "state" rather than a "weight." That "state" is normalization of heart rate, blood pressure, temperature and return to normal social behavior. In girls it also includes return of menstruation or the start of it, and in children category A-C (above) the resumption of growth in height. Rarely can a child who is genetically programmed to be larger than average be safely held at a "thin" body weight. Size acceptance may be a part of the family's treatment challenge.

III. **Group Three: Children who are growth stunted.** These children also represent a special case. Sometimes girls who have been growth stunted for years prior to receiving treatment for their anorexia nervosa have been treated by family and friends as "petite" "dainty" and "elfin." They may like this. Parents may like it or at least accept it. As such children begin to grow both they and their parents may have to re-adjust their expectations of what this child will look like once they are healthy. Look at the family growth patterns, look at the growth percentile along which the child grew before they showed signs of growth slow-down. Do not accept partial treatment. Not only is the body being stunted, but the brain as well.

In summary, what is a young person's ideal body weight, down the line, when they are fully grown? It is the following: That weight (in females) which allows them to have normal ovulatory periods and which they can maintain when not engaged in eating disorder behaviors.

In other words, if the only way a person can maintain a certain weight is by constant restrained eating and exercising for the sake of weight control, then that weight is not their body's ideal weight.

Children need to grow, they need to play, hang out with friends and family, learn and did I mention grow? Don't settle for anything less.

Returning now to the admission criteria:

4. **Refusal to eat or "acute food refusal"** (as we call it in our clinic) is not the same as "refusal to eat enough," which would apply to nearly every eating-disordered patient. It is literally the inability to take in any but the tiniest amounts of food (and sometimes water or other fluids), which would clearly make the induction of re-feeding impossible outside the hospital. If the patient is otherwise medically stable, the inpatient stay can be very brief (the period of time it takes to adjust to a minimum of 2,000 kcals/day), and he or she can then be transferred to the DTU. Usually, however, a patient who has been eating almost nothing destabilizes with re-feeding and needs to stay in until orthostasis resolves. Patients with acute food refusal may very well need to be started out with nasogastric tube feeds. And if so, remember: Tube feeding is not a problem, it is a solution.

5. **Body fat <10%.** At the Kartini Clinic we refuse to measure body fat, because it is just one more number for patients to perseverate on. We do not use it as an admission criterion, but some places do.

6. **Temperature <96 F.** We do not use this as an admission criterion as such, but rather view it within the whole picture

of severity of illness. If the patient has been starved and has this temperature, the likelihood that they will be bradycardic is high.

The AAP distinguishes between admission criteria for bulimia nervosa and for anorexia nervosa, which we do not find helpful, because patients with the purging or binge-purging variant of AN meet the "bulimia" criteria also. As far as we are concerned, our expanded list of admission criteria applies to all three diagnoses (AN, AN-P, AN-B/P, BN) and includes the following guidelines as well:

7. **Syncope.** Not all people who faint belong in the hospital, but eating-disordered patients who do need to be hospitalized and on telemetry (continuous wireless cardiac monitoring) [118]. We do not know how many syncopal episodes (fainting) take place on the basis of orthostasis and how many are asystolic episodes (cardiac arrest). I do know that we have had about a dozen children who have had "asystolic episodes"—where the heart was seen (on the telemetry tracing) to have stopped. These asystolic episodes have lasted 16 seconds with (of course) syncope. Because the patients were young and did not have other underlying cardiac anomalies, they recovered spontaneously, without cardioversion (shocking the heart), but they were down long enough for a code team to be called [64]. And I can tell you that both parents and doctors had a few years taken off their lives by the experience!

8. **Serum K (phosphorous) <3.2 or Cl (chloride) <88.** These blood abnormalities could, in theory, be corrected in the emergency room, but if your child is then discharged home only to continue bingeing and purging, they will just

be back the following night, making such an intervention—at the very least—not cost-effective. I notice the AAP did not include hypophosphatemia (phos. <3.0) since this is usually an artifact of re-feeding and will not occur until and unless the child has begun to eat after prolonged semi-starvation. [64]. We have seen this low drop in phosphorus a few times when a patient or their family has been scared enough by the visit to the doctor or emergency room to go home and begin eating a lot. It can also be seen when bingeing follows restricting. This is one very important reason why it is not safe to advise starved patients to "just go home and eat a lot" [? ]. It is another reason I feel that the *very ill or starved child* should probably not be re-fed at home where monitoring the possible effects of re-feeding is not possible.

A "clinical pearl" for a doctor's or therapist's office: *Never advise a starved patient to go home and eat a lot.* If a doctor is determined to try to re-feed a child as an outpatient and that child has lost a significant amount of weight and has had very low food intake for weeks or months, the doctor would be well advised to check phosphorus levels daily for the first week that they begin to eat and have a plan for replenishing it if it is low. This caution naturally extends to those parents who re-feed entirely at home.

9. **Esophageal tears, hematemesis (vomiting blood) and intractable vomiting** all require inpatient evaluation and the enforced abstinence from purging that a hospital stay offers. On our unit all bathrooms are locked, and patients are not allowed off the floor. It is not enough just to be in the hospital, it has to be a hospital where they have enough experience with eating disorders to know how to structure

the environment so that purging cannot take place. There can be no unsupervised access to the bathroom. It is a safety issue.

10. **Suicide risk.** It goes without saying that a child or adolescent who is at significant risk of suicide needs an emergent evaluation by a mental health professional for psychiatric hospitalization. As a parent, if you are concerned that your child is suicidal, trust your instincts and insist on emergent care. You are the expert in your own child. If you cannot get swift psychiatric attention, your doctor can hospitalize your child with a 24-hour sitter and suicide precautions until a mental health evaluation can be arranged.

11. **Failure of outpatient treatment.** This is the final admission criterion from the AAP, and it makes absolute sense. If you are able to explain this ("we tried a lower level of intervention and it didn't work") to your insurance company, then you have found an enlightened company who understands that hospitalization when outpatient interventions don't work will wind up saving the system money. In fact, in a perfect world, this would be the only hospitalization criterion we would need to discuss. If your child can be safely re-fed by you and your outpatient team, then more power to you. If that has not worked, then be aggressive—and teach your doctor to be aggressive—about getting inpatient care. Just do not wait too long and do not let anyone ignore your concerns.

## 13.2    The Kartini inpatient eating-disorder unit

A perfect eating-disorder inpatient unit would have dedicated beds, locked bathrooms, 24-hour psychiatric and medical nursing, and be physically contiguous with the DTU and other step-down programs as well as the outpatient clinic. There would be a large Ronald McDonald House nearby as well as cheap, safe housing for the parents of young adults; there would be a dedicated school, and more. Even the best children's hospitals (including ours) do not meet all these ideals. Which ones are essential?

When I first began hospitalizing children with AN in our community children's hospital [? ], I experienced all the difficulties inherent in working with a generalist nursing staff who, although very competent, did not understand our type of patient. Additionally, the response to our patients from many other doctors on the ward ranged from puzzled to hostile. The treatment of the patients, when my back was turned, was punitive and often judgmental. The rules were harsh because we felt we could not explain treatment goals adequately to all shifts of all nurses. I felt myself too busy to take the time to train the nurses in the care of eating-disordered patients. Boy, was I wrong! It wasn't until I resigned myself to using my day off to do in-services for the nurses that things got better for us all. Immediately. Every hour I spent in those in-services paid off in years of cooperation, insight, and great nursing care on the part of the pediatric nurses. Once they understood the nature of the illness and the special requirements for their care, they became the children's best allies and advocates. Although the eating-disorder service remains very structured, it became unnecessary to have punitive rules to make the patients cooperate. As soon as hospital staff understood the necessity for it, the hospital placed locks on all the bathroom doors to prevent purging or, much more commonly, surreptitious exercising.

A few years ago our children's hospital instituted Nurse Case Managers for several services, including ours. At first we were not sure we wanted to be "managed," but it turned out to be wonderful. Nurse managers do the day-to-day communication with the insurance companies and are on the floor to field questions and help families when the doctors are in their offices. Additionally they can help families arrange lodging at the Ronald McDonald House when appropriate.

All of our patients have their own room and bathroom (which is locked), most of them are on telemetry (continuous wireless cardiac monitoring), all meals are supervised by a nurse. Once patients are on Phase III (see below), they eat with the other eating-disorder patients in the common room, but always under supervision of a nurse.

A word about the Ronald McDonald Houses attached to many children's hospitals: Never was a charity of more service to families with chronically ill children than the RMcD Houses! The fact that families can afford to stay near their ill child in cleanliness, comfort and psychological support is near miraculous. I would urge all people concerned with the care of children to support their local Ronald McDonald House. It is a gift to families. Just ask those families.

## Summary of essential components to an inpatient service

1. Children's hospital or dedicated children's ward within the hospital.

2. Strong physician advocacy and 24/7 medical coverage.

3. Pediatric nursing care and ancillary services.

4. Case management with the insurance company.

5. Control over the food offered by the hospital kitchen.

6. Ability to monitor strict I&O's (intake and output).

7. Locked bathroom doors.

8. Peaceful, friendly, no-negotiation atmosphere.

9. Telemetry.

10. Access to timely pediatric psychiatric evaluation/consultation.

11. Phased activity protocols.

12. Ronald McDonald House or other low cost or free housing for families.

13. In-house school or tutoring.

**Visitors:** As pediatricians we never separate children from their parents. This rule goes for young adults as well. Where there is significant family strife, we ask that only the primary parents visit (as much as they like) until the family therapist can help make a determination about what will be most helpful to the child as family as a whole. We do not let siblings visit unless the patient requests it. Parents, trying to balance the interests of all their children, are often shocked at how frequently a child does not want their siblings to be allowed in the hospital. We ask the family to respect this and to try not to make the patient feel guilty about this decision, which they often change.

Apart from parents and siblings (and an occasional priest, rabbi, or minister at the family's request), no other visitors are allowed. This means that friends do not visit and neither do grandparents, aunts, uncles, close friends of the family, or others.

Although grandparents care deeply about their grandchildren (I am a grandparent myself) it has been our experience that grandparents and other family members can be a prime source of counterproductive comments which are impossible for us to control. Some common comments we used to hear when relatives were allowed to visit were, "why won't you just eat?" "Don't you know what you are doing to your parents with this behavior?" And, "you need a good trip to a country where people don't have enough to eat." Or worst of all, "I don't understand why they put you in the hospital—you're not that thin. Why, some of the other patients here are like skeletons!" These comments are not only hard on the child, but very hard on the parents who are struggling with all that they need to learn to support their child's recovery. You would be surprised at how many parents express relief at this rule. To accelerate the family teaching, grandparents or other involved family members are encouraged to attend "parent group," which we provide free of charge.

The "no visitors" rule for friends has another basis entirely. We used to let friends visit, until we noticed the strong "secondary gain" we were fostering. When friends came by with flowers, cards, and presents, many kids never wanted to leave the hospital. I tell our patients that we are "creating a bubble of privacy" around them as they go through the re-feeding and medical stabilization phase.

Another privacy issue has to do with the media. I have been asked many times to "do an article" on children with eating disorders, something that might seem to be great advocacy. When, however, we refused to let our patients be interviewed directly or photographed, the reporters quickly lost interest. I feel strongly that this type of media exposure lends a false air of glamour to weight loss. We have a "no publicity" policy on our service. For those children who wish it, we encourage an exchange of letters or cards with friends and family, although we ask the nursing staff to have the parents read them first for inappropriate content (such as "comments" above). Web access is not allowed during this early phase of treatment because of the pro-ANA websites (websites touting AN as a glamorous "lifestyle choice") through which even very young children can learn self-damaging behaviors (see FitDay: Free Diet and Weight Loss Journal at www.fitday.com).

Although we treat our patients with affection and respect, we want their hospital stay not to be entirely comfortable. It is boring, but never painful or punitive. Many of my older patients, in good remission, have told me later that the only thing that has kept them "doing what they have to do" is the fear that they might have to go back to the hospital. There are no phones in the room, just as no friends are allowed to visit, although children whose parents live outside the Portland metro area (about half of all patients) are allowed to speak with their absent parent once a day.

These rules have been instituted entirely for patient safety and to promote a healing atmosphere on our unit. Most parents are cooperative and understanding, but occasionally some are not. An occasional parent believes that rules are only for other people's children. From the beginning they may insist on "special treatment" and are angry that the eating-disorder staff are treating their child "just like everyone else," when it is "obvious" that their child is "special" and "not like the others." Over the years we have had a handful of parents become so incensed when they realized that they, too, would have to follow the rules, that they angrily withdrew their child from the hospital. It makes us sad to see a sick child leave the hospital, but we have had enough experience to know that families with this attitude are unlikely to succeed in achieving coalition with the treatment team, and that when that is the case, the prognosis for their child with a family-based treatment approach is very poor.

Rarely we have a child who has no parents, whom the grand-parents are raising. Such grandparents are treated like parents, with full visiting rights. A situation in which grandparents live with the family and will be doing some of the cooking is a gray area. In those cases, the grandparents are allowed to visit only if they, too, make a commitment to attend family therapy and parent group. They are usually happy to do so.

If you wonder about the necessity for such structure on the eating-disorder floor, consider the situation of a 16-year-old girl who had been transferred to us from another, more traditional, psychiatrically-oriented program. There, adults were mixed with children and she was exposed to several older women who had been ill for a long time and were angry about treatment. She learned from them to be afraid of the staff, who were trying to "control her." The older women showed her how to run up and down the stairs when the staff was not looking. They showed her a way to hide food at the communal table and which bathroom it was "safe" to purge in. Our more structured unit, she told me later, made her angry at first, but only until she realized we meant business and that she would not be allowed to engage in these self-destructive behaviors. Then she was actually relieved.

**Phases and standing orders:** Our patients require a great deal of attention to detail on the part of the nursing staff and eating disorder team. It is impractical to hand-write orders for each admission, and if we ask the house staff to do it, they will not thank us, so we use standing orders. Our initial standing orders were based on Stanford's, although we have changed them so much over the years I don't think Dr. Litt's team would recognize them today. A copy of our orders is included in the appendices, but please remember that we change them periodically. These orders may be copied and used with attribution to Kartini Clinic. Doctors, do not be afraid to alter them. They begin with the diagnosis, the assigned phase, the caloric level, and instructions for orthostatic vitals. They go on to specify the telemetry parameters, the labs, and medication as well as a DEXA scan (bone density test). The hard work of our Nurse Case Managers from Legacy Emanuel Children's Hospital and the floor nurses in helping us revise the phases and orders over the years has been invaluable. They are in constant revision.

In Appendix C, I have also included the details of the "phases" a patient is moved through by the Kartini doctors. Today virtually all patients are admitted at Phase II (medical bed rest) unless they are admitted directly to the ICU (very, very rare), in which case they are placed on Phase I (critical medical bed rest). Almost all patients, and certainly all with bradycardia or prolonged QTc (an EKG abnormality), are placed on telemetry. We do not routinely perform a cardiac echocardiogram for, although as many as 71.4% of patients have been reported to have a silent pericardial effusion, the clinical significance of this finding is not clear [130].

Phase II patients remain in bed at all times; when they need to use the bathroom, they are assisted by the nurse, in a wheelchair. Showers are not allowed. The reason for this restriction is to prevent an even greater increase in calorie burning (metabolic rate) as we begin to re-feed. Our patients are able to burn an amazing number of calories just by jiggling their legs and they chafe terribly at their "exercise restriction." Many parents, who are proud of what a "good athlete" their eating-disordered child is, suffer almost as much at the restriction as the patients do. Here parents and team can get "out of coalition," and we must anticipate this by addressing it openly.

Once children are gaining weight (usually day 3 or 4, but sometimes sooner), have a heart rate that allows them to safely move around (above 40 or so, daytime), and are eating, they are moved to Phase III. If their heart rate is very low (<40 BPM), we put orthostatic vitals "on hold," having learned the hard way that it is possible to induce cardiac arrest with the vagal stress (stress on the vagus nerve that controls, among other things, heart rate) of going from lying to standing when the heart rate is very low. At no point are patients allowed to walk around without accompaniment or to visit other ED patients in their rooms.

As mentioned, a copy of the details of the five inpatient phases is included in Appendix C. Just remember, if your child is put on Phase III from the beginning, they will experience it as very restrictive, whereas if they "graduate" from Phase II to Phase III, they will experience Phase III as "a big improvement" and be much more cheerful and compliant. Phase IV is where most kids focus their aspirations, because Phase IV allows more walking and more movement, but I try to focus them on the Big Step: Phase V Day Treatment.

# Inpatient activities and team members

Right from the start Kartini Clinic patients work with a family therapist. The role of our family therapists, at this level of treatment and well into outpatient care, is different from that of their role in traditional family therapy. Our family therapists are not primarily there to "fix broken or dysfunctional families." Most of our families are highly functional. The role of the family therapist at the Kartini Clinic is to *take the treatment plan devised by the doctors and make it work for this particular child in this particular family.* In some respects this phase of family work is like (idealized) diabetes education. Analyzing how any particular family works together is essential, and the first part of the family therapist's work revolves around helping the rest of the team understand the internal working relationships within the child's own family. The family meets with the family therapist every week throughout treatment.

At our hospital our children are provided *physical therapy (PT)* and *occupational therapy (OT)*, in a group setting when they are on Phase III. Our patients tend to love PT as they love all movement, although sometimes what they need the most is the structuring of leisure time activities provided by OT. Boredom is an oft-cited reason for bingeing and purging. Even those children who do not binge or purge may show an extreme poverty of *non-body-centered* leisure-time activities and interests.

*Art therapy* is a modality we use with great success in the Kartini Clinic. We often prefer it for individual work for very young, quiet, shy, poorly verbal, or closed-off children.

We work hard to achieve a high level of integration between levels of patient care. With the exceptions of the hospital nursing staff, some of the same staff is employed in the day treatment and outpatient units as in the hospital. As soon as hospitalized patients are stable enough to be off telemetry for an hour and a half, we have them attend *group therapy* on the Day Treatment Unit (DTU), where they will meet the milieu therapists. After all, ideally, the hospital is but a stepping-stone to the integrated physical/psychological work that will be done in the DTU. If the patient has taken a part in group therapy on the DTU while he or she was still an inpatient, he or she will be less afraid and nervous about graduating to the DTU.

From the first day of hospitalization we include *parents* in their child's care. They meet weekly with the family therapist and each morning with the physician during morning hospital rounds. Additionally we provide "parent group" weekly as a forum for parents to lend support to each other and to get further questions answered by the staff. This is the parents' time to hear about the treatment philosophy and to ask questions. It is also a time for them to be able to express their fears and frustrations to other parents who are going through the same things. Occasionally, a parent refuses to attend parent group, saying they "do not want to share" their experience with "strangers" whose children, anyway, are "not like" theirs. This attitude unfortunately will cut them off from their greatest source of support and empathy: Other parents.

Some, although not all, children with anorexia nervosa will have other co-morbid or co-occurring conditions [62] such as depression, alcohol use, anxiety disorders [35], or obsessive-compulsive disorder [52]. (The personality disorders unquestionably have their seeds in adolescence, but making such a diagnosis definitively is usually avoided until adulthood.) If the team needs help sorting out these "co-morbidities" (other illnesses or conditions which are also present) we have our psychiatric provider do a psychiatric evaluation. At the Kartini Clinic our psychiatric providers are *psychiatric nurse practitioners* (PMHNPs) and are cherished team members. In the State of Oregon psychiatric nurse practitioners have the same scope of practice as a psychiatrist. Whether an eating-disorder team uses the services of a PMHNP or a psychiatrist—or both—the most important thing is that they be team players. Our psychological colleagues need to feel supported and respected by their psychiatric colleagues.

The Kartini Clinic treats patients from all over the United States, including Alaska and Hawaii and an occasional child from outside the US as well. As is surely clear from our introductory statements, we require the families to be involved; more than once I have been asked to "just treat the child" and return him or her to his or her parents "fixed." It doesn't work like that.

Over the years, we have been impressed and humbled by the dedication of parents doing "whatever it takes" to care for their ill children. Having a child diagnosed with a serious, chronic illness that requires family-based treatment is like having a bomb dropped in the middle of a family. One parent will have to take time off work and stay with their child in Portland, sometimes for months. I remember a family from the big island of Hawaii where the mother came to Portland for three months, patiently attending every parent group. Accordingly, she got a beautiful result. We have many families who drive from five or six hours away, even in winter, worried as they are about their other children, and their jobs (through which they get health insurance, after all). For these families the opportunity to stay at the *Ronald McDonald House* has proven a godsend. For a nominal fee, families can stay there as long as they need to in order to care for their child. And not only is the house located on the hospital campus, but the facilities are every bit as pleasant as those of a finer hotel. I cannot say enough about the dedication of their entire staff, from those who man their phones to those who raise money for their continued existence.

Our patients tend to be accomplished students and care about academics. School teachers, required by the state of Oregon, are provided by the hospital. The teachers are invaluable in calming both parent and child when they begin to worry about "missing school."

## Inpatient re-feeding

Before we begin a discussion of re-feeding, I think it is time to point out that anorexia nervosa is not at all about lack of appetite. People with AN are hungry, very hungry. Not only do patients report this (in retrospect), but scientists studying neuropeptides and satiety in eating-disordered patients have not found evidence for decreased hunger or satiety in AN [51]. Hunger is being suppressed.

Regardless of the length of hospital stay, the most important thing that happens on the inpatient service is the induction of re-feeding. I say "induction," because rarely are we able to keep a child in the hospital until they are 100% of their ideal body weight . Even were we able to do so, psychologically it is preferable to continue the "patterning of ordered eating" in the least restrictive setting possible. But we have to always remember, *without adequate weight restoration we achieve nothing.*

It is not uncommon for us to be asked to take over the care of children who have been seen in another treatment setting who actually lost weight during treatment there. This is scandalous and reprehensible. The entire purpose of treatment is to restore weight *so that the effects of semi-starvation do not compound those of the actual brain disorder.* Again: *If you don't achieve weight restoration, you achieve nothing.*

Our weight gain goal is an average of 0.2 kg/day, and we push calories until we get it. To accept a lower level of weight gain is to unnecessarily prolong the hospital stay. These weight gain goals may be discussed with the parents but are never discussed with the patient, because they would induce tremendous anxiety. I tell our patients from the start that I will not be discussing their weight with them, but that I will never lie. I might tell them that they have or have not gained weight, but I will ignore questions like "Was it a little or a lot?" "How close am I to what you want me to weigh?" And so on. I tell them, "I will never tell you your weight, but I will never lie to you. If I tell you your weight is either up or down, you can take it to the bank." In those cases where I do share weight numbers with the parents, I am firm that they not discuss them with their child. As any experienced eating disorder doctor or parent can tell you, once you mention weight numbers to a person with an eating disorder, you will never be able to induce them to talk about anything else. All conversational roads will lead to this one subject. The desire of a person with an eating disorder to talk about weight, calories, and fat is nothing short of obsessive.

Obviously this rate of weight gain (0.2 kg/day) is the ideal once re-feeding has been in place for a few days. A severely compromised patient may not be started quite so aggressively. At the start of re-feeding, we try to match, or only slightly exceed, the calories we think they have been eating at home, by history. For the overwhelming majority of patients the starting point will be 1,000-1,200 kcals/day. And we *never* allow any fat-restricting.

It is common for our patients to try and refuse to eat anything they feel might contain fat. If they refuse to eat a food item(s) they will be required to make up the difference by drinking a calorically equivalent amount of a 1.5 kcals/ml nutritional supplement. If they cannot bring themselves to do this, we place a nasogastric tube, stop all oral feeds and drip their calories slowly over 24 hours until they feel ready to eat their entire meals. This is *not* punishment; it is support.

Before I admit a child or adolescent to the hospital, as part of explaining the hospital stay to them, I let them know that I will be asking them to choose between three methods of getting their "nutrition": 1) Taking all nutrition as food, 2) no food, just supplement, or 3) "not having to deal with any food or drink" and receiving all nutrition via nasogastric tube "dripped drop by gentle drop," continuously. If they are unable to decide, I tell them that I will decide for them, but in that case it will definitely be choice #3, because that is the easiest. Most children will choose option #1, but you'd be surprised. Some highly distressed children actually prefer the nasogastric tube in order to "not have to deal with food at all." I explain that in the hospital they will choose from guided options, but that if they choose not to eat a particular thing *they are not in trouble*, they will merely be required to drink the supplement. It is critical to let them know that this will not be punitive. It is even more critical to educate the pediatric nurses caring for such a patient that the child is not being defiant if they can't or won't eat, and that they do not therefore need to be scolded or shamed, but that the missing calories should be matter-of-factly replaced. A peaceful, friendly, no-negotiation atmosphere achieves wonders, and we get almost no prolonged food refusal. Everyone eventually eats. Many are relieved to do so.

When it comes to food, our patients know they have no choice. As more than one patient has told me afterward, "It was a relief to have you guys give me no choice so I could tell my eating disorder: 'I wouldn't eat, but they are making me.'" Very young children are especially relieved by this, and I have had more than one actually ask me to repeat daily: "I know you would not do this if you could help it, but I am your doctor and I am making you." It brings tears to our eyes to see the relief in theirs.

As our patients are initially put on bed rest and are being required to eat more than they have for a long time, it is no wonder they are convinced that they are going to get fat! For this reason I explain (over and over) how the body's metabolic rate decreases with semi-starvation ("like banking a fire"), only to flare up wildly as fuel (food) is added and that, for this reason, it will take a large number of calories for them to be able to gain weight at all. This can be confusing for parents as well and we work hard to help them understand that their child will temporarily require many more calories during the early part of re-feeding than they will require once they are weight restored and that their metabolic rate goes into high-gear for a few months before trending back down towards normal.

We do not discuss calories directly with the patient and request that the parents refrain from doing so. Remember: It is not only the patient who may be anxious about "gaining too much weight," but in our hyper-conscious-about-weight society parents can be, too, even under these circumstances.

The absence of any mention of a nutritionist or dietician in this discussion may have caught your attention. Our hospital does have dieticians and they do help us, but we intentionally keep them in the background. Eating disordered patients love to talk about calories, food, grams of fat, and so forth. The may request to "speak to a dietician" for this reason, but our message is that *food is medicine,* and the doctors are 100% in charge of prescribing. In our experience, whenever there is a dietician in the room our patients begin to bargain, becoming anxious about fat grams and demanding that certain foods be left off their menus.

This is unnecessary and unacceptable. The role of our hospital nutritionists is to make sure that the hospital kitchen staff follows the prescribed diet carefully, but they do not write orders or have direct patient contact. I have further found that when dieticians are in charge of writing food orders, the physicians do not learn to do this and hence never have as complete an understanding of re-feeding. From inpatient through outpatient, the Kartini Clinic doctors and nurse practitioners are required to write all food orders and make all caloric adjustments.

A hospital kitchen can be difficult to manage. None are perfect, although our children's hospital[1] kitchen managers have been our stalwart allies. Many hospitals serve food that I thought had disappeared with the 1950s, such as Swiss steak and Jell-O © salad. This is not acceptable for us because, from the first day, we are trying to educate our patients about a heart-healthy diet for life, which means a diet with lots of vegetables and little processed food. We do not fat-restrict; we require all milk to be whole milk and all yogurt to be whole-milk yogurt (whole milk is real milk, after all). If anyone feels nervous about this, I recommend the article "The Soft Science of Dietary Fat" [120] that appeared in *Science*, a highly respected print source for scientists from all over the world. Or more recently, an article describing weight loss, heart health and varying degrees of fat ingestion from the *New England Journal of Medicine* [105]. Every dinner served by us includes a salad with an (olive) oil based dressing as well as cooked vegetables. We have enjoyed a great deal of cooperation from our hospital kitchen administrator, just by having the doctors treat her as part of the team.

---

[1]Legacy Emmanuel Children's Hospital

We hospitalize, on average, about 90-100 children a year and have done so since 1998. Not once have we resorted to hyperalimentation (where children are fed through their veins) and we do not plan to do so in the future. In my view, hyperalimentation has no place in the treatment of pediatric eating disorders; it is expensive and dangerous. Over a long period of time it requires placement of a central line (one placed in a very large vein close to the heart) with attendant dangers of infection. We find that if the patient is very compromised, adequate ability to titrate small amounts of calories (less than 800) can be achieved easily by placing a nasogastric (NG) tube. Placement of an IV line is required at our hospital for all patients on telemetry (constant wireless cardiac monitoring), giving us the ability to give IV fluids if necessary to correct electrolyte imbalances. As soon as the electrolytes are normal, however, free water can easily be added to the NG tube if the patient is unable or refuses to drink.

Hypophosphatemia (low serum phosphorus) is perhaps the greatest danger we face during the initial phases of re-feeding. The adult literature is replete with horror stories of patients with death-defying electrolyte disturbances, but this is less common in childhood as it implies a long and severe course of purging. Restricting calories alone will not give significant electrolyte problems, which is the reason that vital signs are more important than labs on initial evaluation. Naturally, hypokalemia (low potassium), hypochloremia (low chloride), and alkalosis (a shift in pH toward the alkaline) need to be corrected, although abstinence from vomiting along with calorie and fluid repletion accomplish this over time. It is essential that patients with an electrolyte imbalance not have free access to a bathroom, sink, or garbage can.

Hypophosphatemia, on the other hand, is an iatrogenic condition [39], which means it is caused by the doctor [104], as he/she adds calories. It is much like the hypokalemia caused by correcting diabetic ketoacidosis with insulin. In this case it is phosphorus that rushes into the cells, becoming thereby unavailable for cellular energy metabolism (ATP), and causes tissue hypoxia from decreased levels of erythrocyte 2,3 diphosphoglycerate (2,3DPG) [79].

From our standing orders (see Appendix D), you can see that we monitor serum phosphorus every 6 hours for the first 24 hours then daily after that until we are no longer aggressively increasing calories. We increase calories by 200 kcals every 24-48 hours unless so doing induces a precipitous drop in phosphorus [88]. If we see a downward trend in phosphorus, even though we have not yet achieved abnormal status, we often start a packet of neutraphos daily. If the trend continues, we add more neutraphos, up to one packet four times a day. It has been our experience that hypophosphatemia is very responsive to this low level of intervention; however, a patient who is very starved and fragile and presents with severe hypophosphatemia and/or other electrolyte imbalances may need to begin the induction of re-feeding in the ICU, where our intensivist colleagues help us with aggressive intravenous correction, something that cannot be done on the regular pediatric floor.

How long is a patient kept on the inpatient service in the hospital? What is a typical length of stay? These are questions asked us every day by parents and insurance companies. The length of stay, I tell them, depends on how sick the patient was when they were given to us. It never ceases to amaze us that people are surprised that children who were clearly very ill and starved for many months (sometimes years) before hospitalization often need weeks to become medically stable. In our program a patient is kept on the inpatient service until they have become medically stable (defined as the reverse of the AAP admission criteria) and are able to *eat* (not drink) a minimum of 2,000 kcals/day. It is not possible to integrate a patient into our Day Treatment Unit at less than 2,000 kcals/day.

Officially, a reversal of whichever medical instability criteria prompted admission in the first place is what is needed for discharge, but in fact, our DTU program is strong enough that we are able to make a small exception: Patients whose sole remaining instability criterion is early morning orthostasis can be stepped-down to the DTU. Patients who are compliant with a minimum of 2,000 kcals/day food (not supplement) and who are medically stable except for still being less than 75% premorbid weight can also be stepped-down to the DTU at the physician's discretion. The only problem here arises when the patient has much better medical than mental health insurance; under those circumstances, if a very underweight patient is planning on gaining the majority of their weight in the DTU, they may run out of insurance (mental health benefits) before this is possible. In that case it might be better to have most of the weight gain take place in the  hospital setting.

## Labs

On admission we obtain the following laboratory studies:

**Electrolytes:**  Expect them to be basically normal unless the patient is purging or using laxatives.

**Phosphorus:** This is highly likely to be normal on admission but may fall with re-feeding. Because hypophosphatemia is thought to contribute to certain cases of cardiac arrest, and because, when present, it is caused by re-feeding, we follow it very closely.

**Magnesium:** Hypomagnesaemia has been reported in the literature on anorexia nervosa, but I have never seen it.

**Sedimentation rate (ESR):** We obtain a sedimentation rate because if it is high, we look for another reason for weight loss. Our patients have not only low sedimentation rates, but *very low* rates, usually 1 or 2 mm/hr.

**ASO titer, anti-DNA-ase titer and throat culture:** As mentioned before, PANDAS (pediatric autoimmune neuropsychiatric disorders associated with streptococcus) has been described in the acute onset of OCD in children. We have had a handful of children with the diagnosis of "food phobia" who have had PANDAS, were strep positive, and were *cured* with an injection of penicillin. The late Dr. Mae Sokol has studied streptococcal infection and a possible association with childhood-onset anorexia, and although we constantly look for it, we have never had a documented case [112].

**Pregnancy test:** This should be done in all female patients of child bearing age regardless of their menstrual status.

**Urine drug screening:** We screen the urine looking for caffeine and diet pills and only incidentally for drugs of abuse.

**Complete blood count:** We get this, but it is amazing how rare anemia is in patients with anorexia nervosa.

**Liver function studies:** In severely ill patients we see mildly elevated liver function studies, usually in the hundreds. If you see liver enzymes in the hundreds of thousands, you should consider other diagnoses.

**FSH, LH, estradiol:** We get baseline values for these hormones because we follow them later in the outpatient clinic unless and until we have return of regular menstruation [37].

**Thyroid studies (TSH, T4, T3):** We get baseline thyroid studies because hyperthyroidism (too much thyroid hormone) is a theoretical cause for weight loss. We are much more likely to see mildly *depressed* TSH, T3 or T4 in a patient with anorexia nervosa or depression. It has no clinical significance that I am aware of and corrects with restoration of weight and health. An occasional, usually older, patient may actually abuse someone else's thyroid supplements in order to lose weight.

**Cholesterol:** Although not an acute lab value in most instances, I mention this to alert you to the fact that cholesterol levels can be high in patients with anorexia nervosa. Further, a study reported by the Department of Neurosciences at the University of Padua in 2004 showed a negative correlation between total cholesterol and BMI. In restricting anorexics cholesterol levels appeared to increase with a decrease in weight until the weight was so low that the liver was not functioning properly [25]. Cholesterol levels in patients who also binged was even higher. This means that the clinician acutely caring for a child with anorexia should not attempt to correct any hypercholesterolemia with a fat restricted diet, particularly because low cholesterol has been linked to an INCREASED risk of suicidality, self-injurious behavior, and depression in these as well as other patients [67]. Remember whole milk? Don't be afraid.

Other studies:

**DEXA (bone density):** We get a baseline DEXA (bone densitometry) study on all patients, male and female, as it has not been our experience that low bone density is easily predictable based on menstrual history and also because around 9-10% of our patients are male. Osteopenia and osteoporosis are more likely in a girl who has a low estrogen level or a boy with low testosterone levels. The "medicine" to treat this is food. Oral contraceptives or other hormone replacement regimens have not proven helpful in bone restoration, and studies done by Golden *et al.* on alendronate (Fosamax) have proven disappointing [38]. Although poor bones are an outpatient issue and have little acute (inpatient) relevance, they are sobering news for those who say: "Who cares if she doesn't have periods—lots of runners never have periods!"

**MRI:** As mentioned earlier, we have now had a couple of patients who presented to "rule out" anorexia nervosa who turned out to have a brain tumor instead. For this reason, if there are abnormal neurological findings, or if the presentation is atypical, we get an MRI of the brain. The tumors have been brain stem tumors (except for one: Fibromyalgia, the setting of neurofibromatosis), which a CT scan might have missed. It is not necessary for every patient to have an MRI done, only those who present with atypical findings. This is where an experienced eating disorder doctor comes in.

## 13.3   Medication

Over the years of treating anorexia nervosa, bulimia nervosa, food phobia, or (more rarely) selective eating, we have discovered that medication can be a powerful adjunct therapy to re-feeding. But first we try to *give food a chance.* This has been discussed extensively by Dr. Desocio in Chapter 9. The starved brain can imitate depression and even psychosis, and starvation certainly worsens anxiety  disorders. If the patient is able to eat without being overwhelmed by anxiety, we wait for the brain to be re-fed and then see what we are left with before we make a definitive diagnosis. We may elect to start medications of the class called neuroleptics to facilitate the acceptance of re-feeding. Intensive psychological work (instead of medication) is useless at this point, because the brain cannot process it [130].

It is important to acknowledge that there are no medications— allopathic, homeopathic, Chinese traditional, Ayurvedic or otherwise—that carry zero risk of side effects. The important point is to carefully study the risk/benefit profile of each as they pertain to your individual child. Some parents are comfortable doing this research themselves, others will prefer to "trust the doctor." Either approach seems valid.

# 14 Finally my child is eating... what's next?

Once the patient has been stabilized medically and the family is looking at discharge from the hospital, what comes next? This chapter describes the concept of the so-called "Step-down Units" which are sometimes called "partial hospitalization units" or day treatment units (DTU). In them, the child spends most or all of a day with their eating disorder team, but they are home at night and on the weekends. As far as I am concerned, the hospital stay is merely a prelude to the real work of the day treatment unit (DTU). In the DTU true psychological and social restoration begins and ordered eating and family meals are reinforced and consolidated. Once graduated from the DTU a patient at the Kartini Clinic will be seen in the outpatient clinic weekly by their various outpatient providers: Our medical doctor, therapist, family therapist and group therapist.

## 14.1 The day treatment unit

It was a few years after we began to admit children with eating disorders to the medical floor for stabilization and re-feeding that we took a look at our statistics. It appeared that we were able to stabilize between 80 and 100 patients per year. However, a closer examination of these numbers revealed a dispiriting statistic: 40% of those hospitalized needed to be re-hospitalized within a year.

In those days a patient who was discharged from the hospital was seen directly in the outpatient clinic weekly, with no "step-down" care in between.

Then in 2000, in conjunction with Legacy Emanuel Children's Hospital here in Portland, Oregon, I founded the Legacy Day Treatment Unit, loosely modeled on the one I had visited at Stanford University. Because all of our patients at that time were children 17 years old or younger, more than 90% of them had restricting anorexia nervosa or other restricting eating disorders without purging symptoms. The unit was therefore designed for this population only. In keeping with our belief that maximal homogeneity of the DTU groups would give best results, only this population was admitted. This meant that those few patients we admitted to the hospital with bingeing and purging symptoms were not able to be "stepped down" through the DTU prior to entering outpatient treatment. As such children made up only a minority of our patients at that time, this did not present a significant problem.

In 2003 the Kartini Clinic responded to a tremendous need in the community and began accepting a small number of older teens and young adults, 18-21 years of age, for treatment. Our proportion of older teens (16-17 years of age) in the school-aged DTU seemed to increase at about the same time, shifting our demographics away from an overwhelming preponderance of "restrictors" towards a more mixed population, including those patients who binged and/or purged. By now we had a few years of data and could confirm a dramatic trend: The much lower rate of repeat hospitalization within a year of discharge from the inpatient service for those who completed the DTU meant that the DTU was a powerful tool in preventing relapse. But it also meant that an increasing number of our older adolescents and young adults were not able to take advantage of this improved treatment, because our DTU was designed for young "restrictors" only. Imagine the distress of parents whose children were thus excluded from day treatment once they realized how beneficial it could be! The Kartini Clinic founded a second DTU to accommodate this group of children (with purging subtype eating disorders). and in 2005, we joined the two units into one, although maintaining diagnostic separation where possible.

A separate day treatment unit was also founded to treat college-aged youth (18-21) which will be described in more detail below.

Although insurance companies have always treated our DTUs as "mental health" units for the purposes of reimbursement—an approach I tolerated and have come to regret—the primary goals of the school-aged DTU were always medical as well as psychological. They were:

1. Modeling of ordered eating and family meals.

2. Supporting parental control of all grocery shopping and food preparation and teaching children to accept this.

3. Learning techniques to control anxiety.

4. Diagnosing and treating any other co-occurring mental health conditions such as depression, obsessive-compulsive disorder, social phobia, etc.

5. Continuing weight restoration, if needed.

6. Managing medication, if indicated.

7. Working on relapse prevention.

8. Learning to identify their eating disorder as an illness, separate from their "self."

Even when working on strictly medical or physical recovery issues, the power of a strong therapeutic day treatment *milieu* (a term therapists use for the psychological environment of the Unit as a whole) was found to make all the difference to outcome.

## "Step-down" admission to the DTU

Admission to a DTU is said to be "step-down" when a child is admitted there from the hospital. As mentioned in Chapter 12.7, it has been our consistent clinical experience that "step-down entry" to a DTU is in all ways preferable to "step-up" (admission straight from the outpatient setting). Clearly a child who does not need the hospital should not be there, but we call attention to this clinical observation so that those parents whose children do need hospitalization are able to understand that this seemingly dire step actually confers on their child a major treatment advantage by way of a better attitude toward and acceptance of treatment.

I will say it again: If cost/insurance restrictions were not an issue, a starved patient, or one who suffers from sufficient bingeing and/or purging to come to medical attention, would always be started out on the inpatient service for the following reasons:

1. The induction of re-feeding is always much easier in the "no-negotiation atmosphere" of the hospital where the doctors are clearly in charge.

2. It is safer to begin re-feeding where we absolutely control caloric quantities, can record intake and output, and can monitor electrolytes and phosphorus.

3. Nasogastric (NG) feeds are a simple, viable option in the hospital setting when other forms of oral feeding prove too difficult for the child.

4. The seriousness of semi-starvation and its medical consequences are brought home to the child and the family.

5. Initial vital sign measurements done in the doctor's office for the purpose of determining admission to the hospital can understate the actual degree of compromise. For example, bradycardia (low heart rate) can be masked by caffeine ingestion or nervousness. 24 hours of telemetry (continuous, wireless heart monitoring) gives us a more accurate assessment.

6. Syncope (fainting) and orthostasis (cardiovascular instability) induced by re-feeding can be safely monitored.

7. Access to pro-anorexia websites and counterproductive input from friends and others can be monitored and evaluated. And most of all:

8. Children who start out on the inpatient ward, who would otherwise be negative about the Day Treatment Unit, are thrilled to be stepped down to the less restrictive DTU after a stay on inpatient and therefore are much more compliant with treatment, ordered eating, and mental health interventions. When transferred directly from outpatient life, on the other hand, the DTU seems restrictive.

Parents whose child must be hospitalized at the time of their initial evaluation are often shocked and unhappy about this; actually they have been handed the greatest possible gift: The swift and effective rehabilitation of their child. Every day in the hospital is gold in the bank for future care.

The decision about the timing of step-down to the Day Treatment Unit from inpatient is a medical one. But from the beginning of their inpatient stay, once a child is stable enough to be taken out of the hospital in a wheelchair, and off of telemetry, they are taken to our DTU for group therapy. This early participation, before they are fully medically stable, helps integrate them into their eventual "DTU home." They get comfortable with the other patients and with the staff; they can see that the DTU is a "homey" place (compared with the hospital) and that they will have more freedom and do more fun things, such as yoga, massage, guided leisure with knitting (yes, even the boys like this), games, and music. It is their first real opportunity to open up to other people their own age about what they are going through, under the watchful and therapeutic eye of the milieu therapists.

In order to "step the patient down" to the DTU a child must, by definition, be medically stable (a reversal of the American Academy of Pediatrics admission criteria cited in Chapter 11), although in practice, because of the close oversight on our DTU, we are able to cut an inpatient stay short and move the patient to the DTU early under two circumstances:

1. Where the patient is otherwise medically stable and cognitively able to process psychological interventions but still below 75% of their goal weight or

2. Where the patient's sole remaining medical instability criterion is early morning orthostasis.

Patients who meet criteria #1 and #2 above cannot yet be discharged home, because it would greatly increase their chance of relapse and re-hospitalization, but we feel they can be safely stepped down to our DTU.

Patients whose parents refuse day treatment after hospitalization are usually not considered appropriate for our outpatient program, where success relies heavily on the teaching that takes place in the DTU. We long ago decided we serve children best when we refuse to be a part of what we view as inadequate treatment.

## "Step-up" admission to the DTU

"Step-up" admission to the DTU is said to occur when a patient has relapsed while in outpatient treatment and needs a higher level of care or is seen by us for the first time and does not meet hospitalization criteria. "Step-up" admissions to a DTU are harder on the parents and on the team, because the patient will not have had the early structure provided by the hospital. If the patients are angry or resistant, they are harder to contain. It will be possible to control access to food, opportunities to binge or purge, compulsively exercise, and so forth only during the hours they are on the DTU. This makes progress slower, but not impossible.

## The homogeneous milieu and why it matters

The more homogenous a therapeutic milieu is, the easier it is to manage. From the beginning we have never mixed adults and children and strive not to mix patients with restricting eating disorders with those who suffer from bingeing and/or purging disorders for most of their group sessions.

In the early days of medicine, pediatrics did not exist as a separate discipline; children were treated as miniature adults. It is considered one of the great leaps forward in the care of children to have realized that they are not: Children have their own developmentally appropriate concerns, issues, and biology. The concerns of the 19-year-old college-aged young woman with a serious boyfriend (or even husband) are far removed from those of a 10-year-old boy or girl. For this reason we strongly believe in pediatric units for pediatric patients.

Additionally we have a pure "conditions of disordered eating" unit; we do not mix our young eating disordered patients with those who have other serious mental illnesses (such as schizophrenia, ,conduct disorder, or drug abuse, ) as is often the case on general psychiatric units. To my knowledge, we are one of a very few programs that try not not mix those who binge or purge with those who do not. Why is this?

Parents of children who restrict believe that I do not mix these two populations because the "restrictors" will learn bad habits from "the purgers." Nothing could be further from the truth. We do not believe that "restrictors" learn to purge from "purgers." If such behavior were learned, it would have long since been learned at school or on the Web. In fact, those patients with the purely restricting form of the illness and those with the binging and/or purging forms are very different psychologically and behaviorally as I have pointed out before. Purging anorexia/bulimia and restricting anorexia seem to be two (or three) different brain disorders with an unknown amount of overlap [97] [24] [20] [61] [122]. Every therapist who has worked with our patients tells me that these two populations are very different and that the therapists' approach to treatment needs to be correspondingly different.

What we see clinically is that restrictors often tend to be behaviorally over-controlled, rarely do we have to deal with cutting or other impulsive or novelty-seeking behaviors in this group of kids. Such children rarely engage in risk-taking behaviors involving drugs or sex; they are more reluctant to open up about their feelings; they are very self-directed and often excel at tasks where rigid self-direction is an advantage (such as getting good grades in school).

Unfortunately, some children with restricting anorexia nervosa report to us that they "look down" on other eating-disordered patients who suffer from bingeing or purging. Protecting the patients who binge and purge from the harsh judgment of those who do not is a major reason for trying to separate the two diagnostic groups when feasible. It is important that children who suffer from bingeing and or purging have an opportunity to discuss these challenges in a non-judgmental milieu. Additionally, "pure restricting AN" is the norm among very young patients, whereas problems with bingeing and purging are seen more often among older patients. So this diagnostic separation between the two groups often gives us a very desirable, de facto, age separation. Where we have to choose between separating groups by diagnosis or by age, however, age will take precedence.

## Holistic team

It has become a truism to say that the treatment of eating disorders needs a multidisciplinary team, and indeed, it does. But I go one step further to say that it is a holistic approach that is required. By this I mean that the whole child, the whole person, must be addressed for healing to take place. Except perhaps in surgery, where wound healing is still spoken of, the word "healing" has largely disappeared from common medical parlance. Yet it is healing from the ravages of disrupted or erratic food intake and healing from social isolation, sadness, and fear that many of our patients need. For this reason we have put together a team in the DTU from across the spectrum of medical and psychological care that includes many different kinds of practitioners, and we're not done yet!

**MDs/NPs**: We are a medically-based program, and pediatricians and nurse practitioners lead our team. In the DTU they are responsible for reviewing vital signs and prescribing each patient's diet. They lead the team discussions and accept responsibility for transfer between the levels of care.

**Milieu therapists**: Master's level therapists live in the milieu with the patients, they lead group therapy, they eat with the patients, and they spend the day with them as they go from one treatment modality to another. For the duration of a child's day treatment stay, the milieu therapists become the team's most critical role models and de facto "parents." The patients rely on them and usually become very close to them. The bonds of trust that are forged by a talented milieu therapist serve the patients well throughout their treatment.

**Family therapists**: All patients at all levels of treatment within the Kartini system have a family therapist with whom they work. The family therapist is the primary conduit for information between the staff and the parents. To restate: The job of the family therapist at the Kartini Clinic is not primarily to "fix dysfunctional families," as most of our families are highly functional, but rather to take the treatment plan and help make it work for this particular child in this particular family. I repeat the point because this is another critical difference between our approach and that of other clinics who use family therapists. No one is allowed to opt out of family therapy at any level. Families are the core unit of healing.

**Group therapists**: Group therapy is a very important intervention. "Group" is the one place where the patients can be themselves with no doctors and no parents around. There they are interacting in a guided peer group, and "group" is where they really tell us what is going on with them. Group therapy is where they feel safe admitting to throwing away or hiding food, and where they talk about their friends and their daily conflicts. "War stories" about weight, symptoms, and so on are not allowed, and competitive eating disorder talk is stopped by the therapist.

Some children who attend group for the first time from the hospital are often anxious about or even resistant to doing so. They tell their parents they don't want to talk about their feelings to "strangers," a comment parents may take at face value although it is rarely the real source of their anxiety. To the parents' surprise and shock, when we query the patients closely about their concerns, it turns out that they are often afraid they "will be the fattest person in group," a fear expressed by the most emaciated as well as by patients of more normal weight. We address this anxiety directly and openly and point out that everyone else feels the exact same way. It is not a reason to skip group. If the child remains ambivalent about group therapy (or the parents do), some children may try another approach, telling their parents: "I'm not like those other kids." "Those kids," they explain, have "severe problems," whereas they do not. We try to prepare parents for this ahead of time, but because we parents are often eager to believe that our children are not like other children with problems, it can be a challenge. Opting out of group therapy is not an option, however, since normal socialization is an important treatment goal.

**Physical therapy/body works/movement therapy**: Although physical therapy was not initially conceived of as an anxiety-reducing modality, our patients (and their parents) have a great deal of anxiety around "returning to their sport," "getting enough exercise," and "moving fat into muscle." A return to their sport motivates some children far more than a return to normal menstruation or strong bones. The role of our physical /movement therapists is diagnostic (what shape is the patient in after a more or less prolonged period of semi- starvation and medical bed rest?

What sports or exercise have they engaged in formerly that can be considered healthy and not obsessive or "compensatory?") The therapist's role is also rehabilitative, helping the patient return to full activity without injuring themselves, both for those children with osteopenia or osteoporosis as well as for those whose bones are still within the normal range but who have experienced muscle wasting. The patient's belief that these "exercise and shape" issues are being addressed makes physical therapy, movement therapy and body works groups a great anxiety-reduction tool.

**Occupational therapy**: Often scoffed at by those who do not understand it, the role of the occupational therapist is to help our patients structure their leisure activities. Our patients often have a surprisingly difficult time structuring their leisure time. People with restricting anorexia nervosa, who are often obsessively concerned with their schoolwork, are at a loss to imagine creative leisure where they are just "having fun," fun that does not revolve around competition, calories, food issues, or exercise. People with purging eating disorders may have a more imaginative idea of fun, but often need a lot of help structuring their leisure time. Unstructured time (boredom) has probably done more to contribute to bingeing and purging than any other environmental factor [103]. On our inpatient service we use hospital occupational therapy personnel, but in the day treatment units our milieu therapists and school teacher fulfill this role.

**Yoga**: Both yoga and movement therapy offer relief from the intense psychological and sedentary activities of the milieu and are interventions where patients are helped to "feel good in their bodies." They are both adapted by our practitioners to any physical restrictions our patients may have. Although "finding the center" is a yogic goal, yoga at the Kartini Clinic does not include any religious or spiritual practices whatsoever.

**Massage therapy**: We often have a massage therapist on staff, although many of our patients are quite anxious about being touched. They are often disconnected from feelings in their bodies and do not associate their bodies with physical pleasure. Massage therapy can be physically rehabilitating, but we use it largely for relaxation. Occasionally a patient is referred for regular massage therapy for the treatment of constipation or insomnia [50] [18] [98] [23].

**Art therapy**: Many of our patients are quite artistic and relate well to drawing or painting their feelings, rather than expressing them in words. Art therapy works especially well for patients who are not as verbally expressive and for very young children.

**Individual therapy**: A minority of our younger patients are assigned individual therapy. Family therapy and group therapy have been shown to be as effective or more effective in younger patients [99] [21]. College-aged youth need a more adult approach and hence allof them engage in individual therapy.

**Psychiatric services**: As mentioned, our staff psychiatric providers are currently Psychiatric Mental Health Nurse Practitioners (PMHNP)[1] who serve as valued team members consulting with our pediatricians. A child psychiatrist could clearly fulfill this function as well, but for many programs it will prove difficult to hire a dedicated staff member of this background, as child psychiatrists interested in eating disorders are often rare in the community. We have two major requirements of our psychiatric providers beyond their absolute clinical competence: They must be team players and function well within a multidisciplinary team, and they must be available "under the same roof."

---

[1]See the Oregon State Board of Nursing Position Statement online at oregon.gov/OSBN/pdfs/policies/involuntary.pdf.

**Spiritual dimension**: I believe there is a spiritual dimension to human life. However, because of the extreme difficulty of providing any spiritual services that do not conflict with someone's personal, cultural, or family belief systems, we have elected to leave the spiritual dimension of a child's life to their parents. There are no "spiritual providers" at the Kartini Clinic, and our providers come from all possible backgrounds: religious, ethnic, and racial.

**Hypnotherapy and relaxation**: Hypnotherapy as part of both relaxation and recognition of unconscious barriers to the acceptance of healing can be a powerful tool. No one is ever hypnotized against their will or against the patient's wishes.

## The physical plant

We have made the DTU itself as homey as possible. Food is served at a family-style table, set attractively with real plates and utensils (not disposable). The kitchen is within the unit, but off limits to the younger patients, just as the kitchen will be at home. The interior colors are cheerful, and the furniture is comfortable. The yoga teachers need long expanses of bare wall against which the patients can prop their feet, and physical therapy ideally utilizes a dedicated space. Art! Art! Art! Art from the patients and the staff is everywhere.

## Duration of stay

The entire purpose of inpatient and day treatment care is to assure the team and family that patients can function successfully as outpatients, where they will spend the rest of their lives: back at school, with their friends, back in their extracurricular activities, and preparing for the their adult lives. How long a patient stays in the DTU depends on 1) how severe their eating disorder is felt to be, 2) how quickly they and their families absorb the teaching of ordered eating, food-journal keeping and moderate activity, and finally 3) their psychological readiness for outpatient care as determined by the milieu therapists. Looking back over our experience, duration of stay varies widely between patients, but a minimal stay of eight weeks for younger patients and twelve weeks for college-aged youth is about what most people can expect.

## 14.2 The day treatment program for college-age youth

In 2003 we began our first step-down program for college-aged youth. This program is very different from the pediatric DTU as the needs of this age group with their eventual goal of independent living are correspondingly different. In this chapter, I will refer to the college-aged DTU as the CA-DTU.

The CA-DTU milieu is made up of medically stable patients between the ages of 18 and 22 who have at least graduated from high school or are in the last semester of their senior year and find themselves in one of three common situations:

1. Those who have been asked to take a leave of absence from their college or university because the school feels it cannot assume responsibility for an ill, eating-disordered patient.

2. Those whose parents withdrew them from school (or who withdrew themselves) when they returned home over vacation terribly underweight or otherwise too symptomatic to continue at school.

3. Those who are known to have, or to have had, an eating disorder and are about to enter college, but who want to be certain that they are prepared for independent living in order to ward off a relapse of their eating problems while they are there.

We have had a wonderful group of young adults in this program, whose accomplishments would bring tears to your eyes: They have come from Stanford, from the University of Chicago, from Reed College, from the local community colleges, from Georgetown University, from the University of Oregon, from OSU, from Santa Clara University, and so on. In other words, our CA-DTU patients come from all over: Outstanding kids from outstanding schools, both male and female. What they have in common is a desire to learn to live independently despite their eating disorder. Some have had previous treatment, even a lot of treatment; some have had none. The CA-DTU milieu is mixed ("restrictors" and "purgers") because of the small size (six participants) and the very narrow age range.

The CA-DTU is currently structured so that an enrollee can hold down a part-time job or attend some classes locally while participating. It is currently four days a week, although some days are full days and all meals, and others are shorter with the rest of the day dedicated to individual therapy or family therapy sessions. There is also an opportunity to fix meals independently and report back to the staff the following day. A parent support group is available to CA-DTU parents just as it is available to the other Kartini Clinic parents.

The CA-DTU is pragmatically organized and involves learning to grocery shop without perseverating on labels or counting calories or grams of fat, learning to eat at a restaurant with friends, learning to cook simple, inexpensive meals that fit with the prescribed food plan, and accepting a body weight that will allow normal activities and resumption of menses (in women). In short, it is a challenge!

We are proud of our program for young adults, and we are proud of them and their parents. Even though they are legally adults, they are very young adults, and we require the participation of their parents or (very rarely) a spouse. Family-based treatment does not work in a social vacuum.

**Group therapy:** Every day in the CA-DTU involves group therapy, led both by milieu therapists and by other master's-level therapists from the Kartini Clinic. "Group" is their opportunity to talk about their individual challenges and receive support as well as peer feedback. Once our patients are in college, they will have to learn to deal with many, often uninformed, comments from their peers. Group is an opportunity for experienced and well informed "guided feedback."

**Individual therapy:** Young adults have deeply personal issues that either relate to their eating disorder or can affect their ability to achieve remission. Although cognitive behavioral therapy has been shown to be effective with bulimia nervosa [75], it is less clear which individual treatment modalities are effective in aiding people with anorexia nervosa [125]. Some of our therapists offer CBT (cognitive behavioral therapy), DBT (dialectical behavioral therapy), art therapy, and hypnotherapy.

**Family therapy:** Every program at the Kartini Clinic is family based. Even young adults are firmly embedded within their family-of-origin matrix. Parents are still very important! A rare CA-DTU patient will be married and have "a family of their own," but, as their illness is almost certainly of long standing, even these patients need the support of parents as well as of their young spouse. Family therapy and parental participation is an essential, non-negotiable aspect of our treatment in all settings. Family-based treatment has been recently examined closely by mental health professionals across the country, indeed the world, and found to be very important to outcome [69] [110].

**Yoga:** CA-DTU patients spend a lot of time thinking and talking; yoga offers a healthy stretch, a powerful, quiet, body-centered intervention that reduces stress and helps us "find the center."

**Physical therapy:** Individual assessment by our physical therapist helps patients understand where their bodies are in the moment of treatment. It addresses osteopenia/osteroporosis, muscle wasting, upper- and lower-body strength, cardiac strengthening, and so on. Understanding why adequate nutrition is an essential part of total fitness *is* a cognitive behavioral intervention.

**Cooking class:** Cooking class is lots of fun; it involves meal planning, shopping for ingredients, and preparation of simple meals that can be replicated in a dorm or school setting. Naturally, it also involves eating a communal meal.

**Meal planning and grocery shopping:** These things sound simple but are fraught with pitfalls for an eating-disordered patient. Learning to control anxiety about food with careful planning is an important college survival skill.

**The meal plan:** All patients at the Kartini Clinic follow a meal plan that is essential to our treatment approach. It will be discussed in detail in the next chapter.

**Restaurant eating:** Eating in a restaurant without planning how to do it is, as one of my college-aged patients put it, "like taking an exam you haven't studied for." Today's youth eat out much more often than was common in their parents' era. In the CA-DTU patients learn how to join their friends eating out and still get adequate calories. They must also learn to recognize and deal with the anxiety this sort of eating engenders.

# 14.3  Special Issues in the treatment of young adults

The challenge to treating adults, even very young ones, are great. Developmentally, in the case of the 18-21-year-olds, their eating disorder is acting up at a time when they are striving for greater independence from their parents, yet full independence, because of the illness, is not possible. Two pragmatic issues, rarely discussed openly inevitably involve parents beyond just their participation in family-based interventions: Legal issues and cost issues.

## Legal issues

Legal issues arise almost immediately on evaluation for admission to the CA-DTU. Adults can and do refuse treatment. Patients with brain disorders, with mental illnesses, refuse treatment more frequently than other patients, and those with anorexia nervosa, who very commonly may not want to get better (read: "get fat"), will refuse treatment most frequently of all. For this reason, unless the patient convinces us that they are willing to participate voluntarily, we require the parents to get legal guardianship prior to beginning the program. Once the parents are the legal medical decision-makers, the young adult must comply with treatment. Parents take this step reluctantly, which I think any parent can understand. We wish our children to move successfully through their development, not be arrested as young adults and required to be disenfranchised of their adult rights. But sometimes, it is either guardianship or no treatment. And sometimes, once the initial resistance is over, the young adult is actually relieved to be forced to take steps they know in their heart are necessary and are designed to keep them safe. If we can avoid this step, we do; if not, we march on and support the parents in their difficult decision.

## Cost of treatment issues

Cost issues can be very difficult and stessful, which I think any adult can understand. College-aged youth may only have very inadequate insurance through their school. Those parents who have the opportunity to continue to cover their young adults on their own insurance while they are students would be well advised to do so. If you have any choice in the matter of your insurance, read the policy carefully for reference to mental health coverage and do not hesitate to turn to your employer's ombudsman or Human Relations department, if they have one. If double coverage is realistically available to you, get it.

### Clinical pearls

A step-down unit between hospital and outpatient status is critical for the following reasons:

- It consolidates ordered eating.

- Parent education is essential.

- The child forges a close bond with the whole treatment team.

- Psychological intervention can now happen intensely.

- Teaching, teaching, teaching!

- Young adults need their families, too.

# 15 Is anorexia nervosa chronic or curable?

## 15.1 Maudsley and our family-based outpatient care

When I began treating children with anorexia nervosa the term "Maudsley method" was never mentioned. We were doing family based treatment from the first days of the Kartini Clinic when it was almost unheard of. The more we did it, the more convinced we became that there was really no other way to do it. Families, as I have repeatedly said, are not the problem, they are a major part of the solution. A few years ago whispers of "Maudsley method" began to circulate; today the whispers about this pioneering family-based treatment modality have become a hurricane (a welcome one) where parents have decided to take back control of their child's treatment from those who not only would paint parental involvement as a problem, but who would actually refuse to share information about a child with their own Mom or Dad.

But what is the Maudsley method and do I endorse this approach? The Maudsley approach is named after the Maudsley Hospital,[1] a psychiatric hospital in south London, founded in 1907 to promote both physical and mental health in the community. Dr James Locke of Stanford University and Dr Daniel LeGrange

---

[1] See the hospital website at maudsleyparents.org/whatismaudsley.html.

of the University of Chicago, both psychiatrists who treat eating disordered children, write: "The Maudsley approach can mostly be construed as an intensive outpatient treatment where parents play an active and positive role in order to: Help restore their child's weight to normal levels expected given their adolescent's age and height; hand the control over eating back to the adolescent, and; encourage normal adolescent development through an in-depth discussion of these crucial developmental issues as they pertain to their child".

I do endorse the Maudsley approach as described above with some reservations. Perhaps our family based approach at the Kartini Clinic would best be described as "modified Maudsley." After all, I am a physician who treats children with anorexia nervosa and other eating disorders and not a parent of a child with one. Our treatment modalities were developed based on experience with the hundreds of children we have treated over the years, most of whom could not have been treated in an outpatient setting or they would never have arrived on our doorstep. Those children whose eating disorder symptoms could have been "turned around" with intensive work on the part of parents and a therapist coach and who could then have had "the control handed back over to them" successfully, would never have been referred to a specialist clinic like ours in the first place. This is my opinion. The parents of patients referred to us have usually made Herculean efforts to re-feed their own child at home with or without the help of professionals, and they have watched as their child dwindled to a shadow of themselves, withdrawn, angry and sad. They may have also become "the enemy" to their child in their desperate efforts to help. Many report that the scaffolding of their marriages and family life was stretched to the breaking point with the effort of "doing it on their own." Knowing that sometimes parents were successful with this outpatient approach, Maudlsey or otherwise, made them feel even more guilty and desperate. Rather than understanding that anorexia nervosa, like all human illnesses, has a *spectrum of severity of illness*, they interpreted their child's failure to get well as a personal failure. It is not.

This "referral bias," puts my point of view somewhat at odds with the individual experience of any one parent who is working the Maudsley method successfully. Conclusions drawn on the basis of those children who respond to re-feeding at home and then go on to be symptom-free are necessarily different than conclusions drawn on the basis of hundreds of dedicated families whose child's symptoms were either so advanced or so severe that they needed initial hospitalization and close outpatient follow-up to remain in remission. But our viewpoints are—in my opinion—complimentary rather than opposing. We have far more in common, far more, with Maudsley parents than we ever did with practitioners of the older treatment paradigms which focused on removing the child from the "ill family" or which searched for the cause of childhood onset eating disorders within the family. Like Maudsley practitioners we remain agnostic as to the cause of anorexia nervosa and focus instead on the "how" rather than the "why" of childhood eating disorders. We focus on rebuilding a child's life after the ravages of the illness are contained and rebuilding it within the context of their own family.

The majority of our patients will have gone through either our inpatient program followed by our day treatment program or have come through our day treatment program directly; they are all then followed in our outpatient clinic.

When parents are scared and desperate and a child is in the hospital, hospital and DTU seem to be the most important steps in achieving remission and, indeed, they are very important. But it is outpatient follow-up that is critical to long-term success, to long term remission. "Outpatient" is where the child will be returned to school, to their friends, to their homes. It is where everything they have learned in DTU will now be applied.

In the past, we have seen many children sent off to residential treatment centers, most of which do not have outpatient programs. Parents are encouraged after residential treatment by "how good the child looks" and are too weary to fight with their child about the need for further follow-up. After thousand of dollars (as much as $160,000 as of this writing for which families may have mortgaged their homes) and months of intensive residential treatment, we have watched as children slowly relapse in the community. But now the family's resources have been depleted and their will to fight diminished. Discharge is usually to a "local team," almost invariably their family doctor, a nutritionist, and a therapist. Communication from the residential treatment team to these providers consists (at most) of a ream of paperwork from their residential stay, *perhaps* a phone call from one of the residential therapists (rarely a physician). By design, the residential therapists no longer communicate with the patient. This waste of resources when the child relapses is a terrible shame and could have been prevented by spending the same energy developing firm outpatient resources as was spent on residential resources. It is as if you had major complex surgery and were returned home with general care instructions but your treating doctors had no further interest in your recovery, refused to see you or talk to you and merely sent you off with vague instructions to "see someone in your community."

But what does *adequate follow-up* mean and for how long? Which providers are essential and for how long? When do we return our patients to their pediatricians or family practitioners? How long? How long? This question now becomes the focus of the family's energy. They have endured agonizing weeks, months, or sometimes years of watching in frustration and fear as their child wasted away or binged and then got rid of good food by vomiting, and they have gone through the challenge of finding adequate help followed by the intense experience of hospitalization and day treatment. They are now "ready for it to be over." How long?

From the beginning of treatment we stress two things: The *chronic nature of anorexia nervosa* (see discussion below) and the *spectrum of severity of illness*. What does this mean? It means that "how long?" is an unanswerable question; it means that the goal is *remission* and that the length of time the patient spends in remission depends on adequacy of treatment, parental unity with the team, and—of course—severity of illness.

At the time of graduation from our day treatment unit, I meet with the parents and explain to them that while outpatient treatment is less intensive than the hospital or day treatment, it will still require many visits and almost certainly will interfere with school. It is important to stress this right up front because many of our patients (and their parents) are very achievement-oriented and anxious about their child "getting behind." Missing school is unfortunate, but not nearly as unfortunate as relapsing and suffering another trip through the inpatient service or as unfortunate as experiencing a lifetime of chronic illness and social withdrawal. In our experience, if the eating disorder is not adequately addressed during the school years, it will crop up again at the end of high school or during the first years of college, and then it will cause real academic failure.

As our patients move through their outpatient treatment and do well we will begin to see them less frequently, at first weekly and then every two weeks. After about three or four months of follow-up, if they are doing well, we graduate to monthly visits.

Once they have been able to remain successful for 3-4 months at a level of monthly follow-up, they are usually graduated back to their family physician or pediatrician. But before they are graduated they will do something important in family therapy: The parents will draw up a list of symptoms that they agree would prompt a return to treatment, no argument needed. They get a copy, their child gets a copy, and we get a copy. This idea is relatively new and one we hope will result in earlier recognition of relapse, should it occur.

The child also draws up his or her own list titled: "What would it take to convince me that I need further treatment," and parents are given a copy.

## 15.2   Is anorexia nervosa a chronic illness?

Recently, while responding to a struggling parent who had posed a specific concern on the *FEAST website* (http://www.feast-ed.org) I used the word "remission." Another mother on the forum responded that she did not like my use of the word "remission" since she preferred to think her daughter's illness was not chronic. Until that moment it had not occurred to me that this question of chronicity was a controversial one for some parents.

Ken Nunn, neuro-anatomist, eating disorder specialist and great thinker, wrote an important chapter called "The Sensitivities that Heal and the Sensitivities that Hinder" in Drs. Lask and Bryant-Waugh's *Eating Disorders in Childhood and Adolescence 3rd Edition.* In it Dr. Nunn called childhood anorexia nervosa a "malignant disease of children with parents usually trying to do more than could be expected of any parent..."

"Malignant disease" puts it well and, as one who has tried to help families come to grips with early onset anorexia nervosa, I echo this description. Anorexia nervosa has the same lifetime mortality rate as some types of leukemia (and we don't stop loving and being terrified for our children just because they become young adults). The spectrum of severity of illness in anorexia nervosa is very wide, with some people whose illness is so severe that they lose their lives to it while still young; some are unable to conceive children later in life or to care for those they have; some have less severe illness with periods of complete quiescence and there are even some cases where symptoms mysteriously disappear and seem to be gone forever. But all children can be treated and most can be treated successfully.

What are the patterns we observe with this disease when it strikes in childhood and adolescence? Does it rise up suddenly, get treated and disappear? Does it creep up on the patient and family, then respond to treatment? Does it seem to go away and then resurface in times of stress or change or for no apparent reason? There is definitely more than one pattern, so let me try to describe what I have seen over the course of more than 1,500 children with eating disorders, more than 80% of whom have anorexia nervosa or one of its variants.

Anorexia nervosa can begin abruptly or appear to do so. It can also start slowly, or appear to do so. Often the signs and symptoms get ignored or glossed over, more often by physicians than by parents, but sometimes by parents as well. No one wants to look for trouble. Everyone wants their child to be "normal," for everything "to be alright." Commonly, in retrospect, our patients tell us that their preoccupation with weight/fat/food or similar began long before any physical symptoms of the illness appeared, sometimes many years before. Some children remember having a personal, unspoken concern for these issues as far back as earliest childhood.

When I first began treating childhood eating disorders, adult providers often spoke of "recovery," a term borrowed from addiction science. I did not feel that it rang true for our young patients. Over the ensuing years of following our patients, the chronic nature of anorexia nervosa began to strike me. It acted like so many other diseases of "remission and exacerbation," chronic conditions such as depression, anxiety, diabetes, rheumatoid arthritis or inflammatory bowel disease. It was clear that anorexia nervosa could seem, for all intents and purposes, to be gone only to reappear (or to try to) after months or years. There seemed to be no distinct way for us to predict the course, although a common resurgence time was late high school or early college. Some cycles were shorter: Six months of good health where the eating disorder seemed to be gone only to resurface with increasing ED thoughts for a few months and then to remit again with more treatment.

I began to think in terms of "relapse" and "remission." Why? For me these were hopeful terms—and more importantly, they were honest terms. How does it serve a family for us to imply that their daughter or son has been "cured" when this flies in the face of our own clinical experience? Even if you are very uncomfortable telling parents what no one would want to hear, does it make sense, is it fair, to give them this (often but not always) false hope and let them find out the truth on their own? For find it out they will. My concern is that if we frame a child's condition as "cured," when they do relapse the parents will experience this as a personal failure—either their own or the child's. It is not a failure, not even a treatment failure, it is the nature of the illness. Understanding that we do not cause and therefore cannot "un-cause" is both empowering and terrifying. As parents and providers we offer up all of our strength, resources, love, knowledge and the power of good medicine and food. More we cannot yet do, given the state of the science. Usually, it will be enough to get young patients into remission and to allow them to grow and develop normally while their brains heal.

Can anorexia nervosa ever spontaneously remit? It can. Is that the usual pattern? No. Can it "disappear" with treatment and never come back? It can. But that is not the usual pattern, anymore than it is usual for the other above-referenced chronic, medical and psychiatric conditions of childhood.

By focusing on the relapsing nature of the illness we can de-stigmatize the journey. Of course, at first parents are saddened (even angered) to learn how long the road will be. Who wouldn't be saddened? But if they can be bolstered by the near certainty of achieving a happy and successful life for their child, is not the truth better? Let's honestly recognize the illness for what it is: A potentially malignant disease of childhood that can be firmly brought into good remission and which, when it relapses, can be brought back into remission with the tools we have learned to use.

So, is anorexia nervosa a chronic condition? It usually is. But this chronicity does not reflect poorly on the child, the parents or even the treatment team. It just is the way it is.

Ken Nunn ends his chapter with these words: "But AN is not immortal any more than smallpox or poliomyelitis. It is time to systematically, tenaciously and strategically seek a cure, just as our colleagues in oncology seek a cure for the malignancies they face... There is much we can do today that even a decade ago we could not have achieved. There is much more we could do if all those who suffer or have loved ones who suffer combined forces with clinicians to "crack" this malignancy of mind and body. There is so much more suffering that could be relieved by the simple recognition, by the community as a whole, that those who suffer with anorexia nervosa should be accorded the same dignity as those who suffer with other malignancies. The dream of healing anorexia nervosa will only be realized at a very substantial cost; the cost of us as a community becoming aware of the pain of those who suffer from anorexia nervosa, the anguish of those who care for these young people and our responsibility to relieve their suffering and anguish."

There are unquestionably children who experience a "bout" of anorexia nervosa that remits with treatment and then seems to go away "for good," with a complete return to normal eating and activity. But this, in my experience, is not the norm. Most patients are able to achieve remission of most of their symptoms and learn to control and redirect their persisting eating-disordered thoughts, but will relapse during periods of stress, growth, change, illness, or for no apparent reason. I submit that this is typical for most chronic disease of man. Lupus, rheumatoid arthritis, inflammatory bowel diseases, and others are well known to worsen with stress, illness, or for no apparent reason. The question for most patients is not "Will they relapse?" but "How do we recognize relapse early and get them back into remission promptly?"

So let's not despair—far from it—but fight on.

Below I will go into more detail about the various outpatient interventions we recommend, followed by a discussion of the most common outpatient issues: Return of menstruation, fat re-distribution, and control of weight gain.

There can be no one "recipe" for outpatient care; even within the Kartini Clinic we are constantly working on and improving our outpatient approach. But now it's time for me to talk about the single most important intervention we have, and also the most controversial: The meal plan.

# 15.3   The Kartini clinic meal plan (KCMP)

The Kartini Clinic meal plan grew organically over time out of the need for our patients with all conditions of disordered eating to achieve some balance in their lives and some quiescence to their symptoms. Whether those symptoms were restricting, bingeing, or purging they had chaos and irrational food fears and beliefs at their core. We needed a plan for ordered eating that would "pull the rug out from under" skipping breakfast, sometimes lunch and snacking ravenously or raiding the refrigerator in the afternoon or evening, followed by intense guilt and compensatory behaviors of one type or another (e.g. exercise, purging, cutting). We also needed a meal plan that children who primarily just restricted their intake could come to accept, one that would reduce their intense anxiety but also promote good general health and growth and was culturally acceptable. We emphatically did not need "a diet."

Over the years many young patients have told me that the meal plan was the core intervention that allowed them to heal, then trust and finally stay in good remission. But publishing our meal plan on the web created an unexpected firestorm of criticism from Maudsley parents. Many of them were concerned that a meal plan that did not include fast food or sweets was ridiculous and "not realistic." They wanted their kids to "eat normally like other kids."

Let's be clear: Children who have anorexia nervosa are—for better or for worse—not like other kids when it comes to food. I would like to see this be "for better." It is true that patients on our meal plan eat a healthier diet than "normal" or "average" kids do, but why would you object to that? Would you object if they were smarter than normal or average, or got better grades? It is true that we require family meals, cooked and eaten at home, but I submit that if this is not "the norm," it should be.

A copy of our meal plan is included below along with a general discussion of its utilization. By following our meal plan we not only assure weight restoration, but also avoid the common problem of gaining too much weight once weight goals have been achieved.

I want to begin the discussion of our meal plan with some salient points before I go into the details of why we do things as we do:

1. The Kartini Clinic Meal Plan (KCMP) was developed to enable families to feed their children *without resort to counting calories or exchanges*. The child chooses among real food items that have been counted already (by us). Many different food choices are available.

2. Within the confines of the meal plan (KCMP) parents can cook traditional American food, if that is what their family likes, or Chinese food or Indian food or Russian food or German food, Nouvelle-cuisine, French food, Japanese food...you get the picture.

3. It *is* true that our meal plan does not support fast food.

4. It *is* true that we want parents in charge of the food: Purchasing food, cooking meals, setting aside time, as a priority, to eat as a family.

5. It *is* true that we don't allow low-calorie, low-fat, or diet options or drinks.

6. It *is* true that we require daily family dinners (not a problem for some, a big adjustment for others) and parents to record what their eating disordered child eats at each meal.

7. It is *not true* that our patients must stay on the meal plan (KCMP) forever. In fact, at one year after the onset of re-feeding we sit down with the family of a child who is doing well and ask ourselves: "Should we stop recording what is eaten?" "Is it time to add desserts or other treat items, etc.?" "Should we continue to write down what is eaten, but eat without restriction?" If they have already graduated from our program we urge them to ask each other the same questions.

8. It is *not* true that the meal plan is rigid; it is limited only by a cook's (parent's) imagination. You can serve meat, nuts, milk, yogurt, kefir, cottage cheese, cream cheese, chicken, fish, tofu, eggs, French toast, homemade pancakes or waffles, olives, beans, cheese, olive oil or any other oil, ghee, butter, mayonnaise, bread, pasta, rice, bagels, granola, cereal, grits, couscous, quinoa, potatoes, sweet potatoes, cornbread and every imaginable vegetable and fruit, to name a few. You can even serve pizza with a big vegetable-y salad and full fat dressing, as long as pizza doesn't become all that you serve or all that your child wants.

9. The time to leave the meal plan behind is very variable and individualized to a child's progress and age.

The food plan (shown in Figure 15.1) is the blueprint for what we, at the Kartini Clinic, call ordered eating. Ordered eating is the cornerstone of both physical and psychological recovery from

NOTE:    TSP= teaspoon; **TBSP**=tablespoon; **1 TBSP**= 3 TSP

| | Place & Time | Food and Liquid -- AMOUNTS | Parental signature |
|---|---|---|---|
| **BREAKFAST**<br>1½ c. cereal or 1 c. oatmeal<br>1 c. whole milk<br>2 eggs<br>**OR**<br>2 pieces toast or large bagel<br>2 TBSP butter or 2 TBSP peanut butter or 4 TBSP cream cheese<br>**OR**<br>1 c. granola and 1 c. whole milk<br>**OR**<br>French toast:  2 pieces whole wheat bread, 2 eggs, 1/3 c. whole milk, ½ TBSP butter<br>**AND:**    1 Piece of fruit (in addition to above choices)<br>ADD ONS: | | | |
| **LUNCH**<br>**Sandwich**: 2 pieces bread with<br>4 oz turkey/chicken/beef/ham or 3 oz tuna<br>with 1 oz cheese or 1 TBSP mayonnaise<br>**OR**<br>5 TBSP tofu  pate<br>**OR**<br>2 boiled eggs and 1½ TBSP mayonnaise<br>**OR**<br>2½ TBSP peanut butter, 1 TBSP jelly or jam<br>**OR**<br>Grilled Cheese: 2 pieces bread, 2 oz cheese, 1 ½ Tsp butter<br>**AND:**    1 Piece of fruit | | | |
| **SNACK**<br>6 crackers, 1 oz cheese, 1 piece of fruit<br>**OR**<br>One 8 oz whole milk yogurt<br>ADD ONS: | | | |
| **DINNER (WITH FAMILY)**<br>4 oz chicken/fish/beef/pork **OR** 8 oz tofu **OR** 2/3 c. beans with ½ oz cheese **OR** 3 eggs<br>**AND**<br>1 c. cooked pasta/rice **OR** 1½ flour tortillas **OR** 3 corn tortillas **OR** 6 oz potato **OR** 2 pieces bread<br>**WITH**<br>1 TBSP butter/olive oil **OR** 4 TBSP sour cream **OR** 1 oz. cheese<br>**AND**<br>1 c. salad<br>1 TBSP dressing<br>1 ½ c. fresh, cooked vegetables<br>**AND**   8 oz whole milk<br>ADD ONS: | | | |

REMEMBER:  PLEASE BRING YOUR FOOD JOURNAL TO EVERY VISIT.  PATIENTS WITHOUT A FOOD JOURNAL WILL NOT BE SEEN.   NO DIET, LO-CALORIE, OR LIGHT FOODS/DRINKS.

**Figure 15.1:** The Kartini Clinic Meal Plan (KCMP).

anorexia nervosa because it is as much about anxiety reduction as it is about adequate nutrition.

The core importance of the meal plan can hardly be overstated. *Structure* in the treatment of disordered eating is the critical, yet oddly most controversial, part of our treatment program. Let me make it clear: The meal plan is not important because I care what our patients eat, but because they do. Ordered eating is the single greatest (natural) medication we have to control anxiety while achieving necessary weight goals.

In its highest form our meal plan is loosely based on a Mediterranean diet, with an emphasis on fresh vegetables, olive oil, and reasonably small amounts of meat or fish. For those American parents for whom "Mediterranean diet" sounds foreign and unattainable, the KCMP can be used to create a more "normal" American diet or adapted to fit dinners such as stir-fry, tacos, burritos, or even barbecue, although it always requires fresh vegetables and a daily salad. Making your own salad dressing is incredibly easy, cheaper than buying it and more healthy. This might be difficult, but do the best you can.

Basically our meal plan is compatible with most styles of cooking except one: Cooking based on casseroles. Some of my parents have jokingly referred to this as their "church food" and, indeed, it has proven a challenge for families whose social functions revolve around communally served food such as lasagna, tamale pie, noodle casserole, and so forth. There is nothing necessarily wrong with this style of eating, although it is often based on canned ingredients rather than fresh ones and may be heavy on the saturated or trans fats because of a preponderance of hamburger, canned soups or sauces, but the main reason we do not encourage it is because it presents a giant "math problem" for the parent whose child is eating according to the KCMP.

Depending slightly on the actual choices made, the KCMP represents 2,150 kcals/day, sufficient for a teenaged female who is not particularly active. Boys require more calories, children under 11 years slightly fewer. The fat content of the KCMP will be less than 30%, as "heart-healthy" as the parents choose to make it (our recommendation would be for frequently choosing olive oil as the fat source.) This is the baseline meal plan. If more calories are needed, they will be added by the physician, initially in the form of whole-milk yogurt or whole-milk yogurt and Benecalorie ⓒ or occasionally Boost Plus ⓒ or Ensure Plus ⓒ. Once a child is in the outpatient clinic and stable, more calories may be added in the form of patient-preferred (though not prepackaged or "fast") foods at breakfast or dinner. Lunch is intentionally small as it is not a supervised meal, in contrast to all the others, and represents, therefore, "endangered calories." Breakfast, snack and dinner are supervised by a parent.

I am often asked why our "add-ons" are in the form of yogurt and Benecalorie ⓒ or (more rarely) Boost Plus ⓒ or Ensure Plus ⓒ, since these are clearly not "natural" foods. The reason is simple, during that period of hyper-metabolism discussed in the chapter on inpatient care, which almost all children experience, a child will need many more calories than they will need once their metabolic rate returns to normal. To cover this increased metabolic need and yet not resort to "hyperpalatable foods" such as ice cream (see discussion below), we use these temporary foods which are easy to add on and *easy to remove*. For athletic girls or boys who may always need lots of calories even when their metabolic rate returns to normal, we eventually replace the "artificial food" with real food choices.

It is difficult for the average person (or medical practitioner) to understand the anxiety that food causes an eating-disordered child.

It is this anxiety that leads to the symptoms we spend so much time combating: Restricting, purging, compulsive exercise, and so on. The anxiety *must* be controlled. When a child is admitted to the hospital, it is because outpatient interventions designed to help them gain weight or control bingeing and purging have not worked.

Our treatment paradigm requires that the patients accept re-feeding. Why do they accept it? Because they have no choice and because I tell them, "I will not let you get fat," and *I mean it.* This means that, despite pressure from parents (yes, it happens) or even from the children themselves, I will not build hyper-palatable foods into their meal plan. Nor will I allow the parents to cheat and "sneak in" extra food. Their meal plan will be designed to return them to a functioning, healthy weight and *not any more.* They come to know that if they are eating on the plan, they are safe from excessive weight gain. That feeling of "being safe" is essential. It is a contract our team has with our patients. "Eat the meal plan and you will not accidentally or inadvertently over-shoot the mark." Eat the meal plan and you will not be required to eat anything in addition. Eat the meal plan and we will insist that your family not require you to "branch out" until you are ready.

One of the most unexpected learning experiences for us has been how dearly many patients cling to the meal plan. The meal plan is started in the hospital, followed exactly in the DTU, where the parents are trained in using it, and adhered to in the outpatient setting. This high degree of continuity and structure is what works, yet some adults see this structured eating as "not normal" or "boring;" they are anxious for their child to "get beyond it." Of course, how boring it is depends on how imaginatively they are cooking within its confines, but the patients themselves are rarely bored, thriving as they do on the *predictability and structure* of the food. One day almost all of them will "get beyond it," but for now, in the first year of treatment it is a powerful tool.

The patient's food journal is reviewed by the physicians and family therapists in our clinic at every outpatient medical visit, and changes are made if necessary. Again, we do not use dieticians for this because their level of expertise is really wasted on something so basic and because I think our doctors need to have a ground-level understanding of what their patient's eat. I have often called other eating-disorder doctors and asked about a referred child's calories and dietary plan only to be told, "Oh, I'm not sure, our dietician does that." This, in my view, is unacceptable.

Finally, after many years of battling for the acceptance of weight restoration as the cornerstone of treatment, we find ourselves able to convince insurers, other physicians, and parents that weight restoration is so critical that they can accept whatever means necessary to get there: Nasogastric feeds, supplements, no-choice oral feeds, parental supervision of and participation in all meals. This acceptance, though, lasts *as long as the patient is in the hospital.* It's when the patient enters day treatment and especially once they graduate to outpatient care that wishful thinking enters the picture in a big way: "She looks so much better, why can't we let her eat normally now?"

"Eat normally" usually means "eat whatever she wants," and parents are thrilled to see an appetite that includes ice cream, cookies, frappuccinos and the like. Yet Ancel Keyes, as discussed in the chapter on human starvation, in his seminal study of starvation in humans, warned us what happens when *ad lib* ("as you like") re-feeding is offered a person recovering from starvation: They will gain too much weight. He also noted that this "over the mark" weight gain eventually normalizes after a few years—but try to explain *that* to an eating disordered child who has trusted you with their weight restoration! To repeat this controversial point: There are no desserts or sweets on our meal plan for the first year, not because there is anything wrong with desserts or sweets, but because these "hyper-palatable foods" as the food scientists call them, encourage—even trigger—overeating during the early phases of re-feeding.

When your child is in the hospital being weight-restored, their food plan is the floor beneath which they cannot fall; in the outpatient setting it is the ceiling above which they cannot rise. Our patients would not trust us if we restored their weight and let them keep going up and up. It would not be fair or healthy—yet restoring eating disordered children with *ad lib* feeds is common. If you have doubts about this, scan a parent web forum (such as the FEAST forum) and you will find entries from parents who are struggling to deal with this effect (excessive weight gain and snacking) once their child has been weight restored. It's scary.

For patients who struggle with bingeing or purging, ordered eating (eating enough fat and calories to achieve satiety at predictable times, starting early in the day) will help prevent binge eating, craving and consequent purging. In the world of eating disorders, we also know that hyper-palatable food items definitely make up the universe of binge foods [72].

Many college students who have left our program for independent living tell me that "the Meal Plan" has been their salvation. They fought against having to follow it when they were younger, but they lean on it now and it helps calm their anxieties about regulating food and weight when they are far from home. Patients this age shop and fix their own food, of course, as that is appropriate for their developmental stage. Getting to this degree of independence is addressed in the chapter on the college-aged DTU (CA DTU).

To summarize, our patients who are in the hospital follow the KCMP guidelines once they are able to eat at least 2,000 kcals. They then follow it absolutely in the DTU and in the outpatient clinic for the first year. The KCMP base calories are 2150/day: Three meals and one afternoon snack. We do not endorse "small, frequent meals" as we do not want our patients to be spending the entire day either thinking about what to eat or engaged in eating (how eating disordered is that?) All dinners are family dinners, parents do the grocery shopping and the meal preparation. Kids need to busy themselves with doing well in school, building lasting friendships, exploring their environment, helping with family chores and finding out what their life interests are. They do not need to pay the mortgage or feed the family or themselves. Food on the KCMP is pretty much what Michael Pollan so succinctly called "real food, not too much, mostly vegetables." It uses only full fat options, no diet/lo-cal etc. Total percentage of fat is a bit under 30%, depending on choices. It can be made to look like a regular American diet with peanut butter and jelly sandwiches, cereal for breakfast and steak for dinner, if that's what you like, or it can be Chinese stir-fry, Italian pasta, Russian, German or absolutely "gourmet," but it cannot be fast food. And when I say real food, I mean real food, made from real ingredients at home and eaten in the company of people we love.

Following a meal plan brings order and predictability to the life of a child with anorexia nervosa. Once parents adjust to the structure of preparing meals at predictable times and supervising them as they eat alongside their child, our children are almost always compliant and relieved. When there is no parental ambivalence about the meal plan the eating disorder finds no "cracks in the system" through which to torment the child with illusions of "choice." There is choice, of course, to the KCMP, but it is definitely guided choice.

Many young patients with anorexia nervosa manage their anxiety by eating the same thing every day. This is fine. Compared to starving, it is a home run and should be seen as such. Give food a chance! Rather than be concerned about "when they might be normal," try to relax into ordered eating and work on achieving normal physical growth and social development as your first year's goal.

Dessert comes later. Didn't your grandma tell you that?

## 15.4    Outpatient interventions at the Kartini clinic

### Medical visits

Medical visits in our clinic are done by our pediatricians. Their job is to review the food journal, which is a record of the child's adherence to the meal plan and which the parents keep if the patient is under 18 years old. We spend a lot of time making sure the parents and child understand the rationale behind careful adherence to the KCMP (adequate weight gain, anxiety reduction, prevent bingeing), and we check weight and vitals. In very young patients growth (height) also needs to be monitored. In female patients who are old enough, return of menstruation needs to be a focus of successful treatment (see discussion below). A yearly repeat of an abnormal DEXA scan for those children with osteopenia or osteoporosis may be needed.

The Kartini Clinic is a multidisciplinary team, but the medical providers are "first among equals" and are expected to set the tone for treatment and be in charge of the overall plan. Nonetheless, no one is allowed to "just see the doctors." Healing of the whole person will not take place if this is allowed.

## Family therapy

If you have read this far in my book, you know that we feel that the treatment of children and young adults will not be successful without a family context within which healing occurs. To repeat: From the very first interview with a new family we include a family therapist who will follow them from inpatient through the day treatment and into outpatient. The role of the family therapist at the Kartini Clinic encompasses more than the traditional one, although they are all qualified to do traditional family therapy. At the risk of repeating myself yet again, their primary role is to *take the treatment plan designed by the doctors and make it fit this particular child in this particular family.* Beyond this, they will also help the family identify stressors within and upon the family that hinder treatment success.

Although we do not believe that there is an "anorexogenic" family or parent, the range of family functioning that the therapists encounter is very wide. At the one extreme are parents who have respectful, harmonious relationships with each other, a two-parent family, adequate financial resources, and an overall healthy relationship with their child; and at the other we find acrimoniously, even violently, divorced parents who hate each other and have dysfunctional relationships with their child as well as severe financial stressors. Naturally, most families fall somewhere in between these two extremes. We have single-parent families, two-parent families, gay families, traditional families, religious families, atheistic families, reconstituted step-families—in short, the full range of families you would see in a general pediatric practice. What we have found, however, as discussed elsewhere, because there is a strong genetic component to anorexia nervosa, is that it is quite common to have more than one affected first-degree relative within a child's family, often a parent. This is discussed further under therapeutic challenges below.

Issues surrounding weight, body size, and shape are fraught with emotional content in our society, and perhaps every society. How a person feels about these things depends on their own size and shape compared with what they perceive as "the norm," on their age, their gender, their family of origin's attitude, and their socioeconomic status (with higher body weight in women being *absolutely* unacceptable in the upper socioeconomic classes in this country and many others). It is quite common for the talk around American family dinner tables (if there is a family dinner table) to be about everyone's weight, diets they are on, apologetic comments about their food choices, and how much they work out. This is very distressing and potentially triggering to an eating-disordered child and needs to be addressed over and over again in family therapy. The fact that we are asking families not only to return to the family table, but also to cook real food for their children and for each other, can stir up a lot of resentment. Balancing the demands of life is hard enough. This requirement is also likely to bring up "division of labor" issues between the parents. Additionally, many eating-disordered children have become the "family chefs," cooking for and feeding everyone else, and the family may have become very comfortable with this state of affairs and resist changing it. Treatment can be time-consuming and lengthy, requiring that the needs of other children in the family be set aside to address the needs of the eating-disordered child. Similarly, resentment, psychological and even physical distress has been reported in the siblings of children with cancer [48] [4], trauma, and other severe illness [107]. Parents need the help of their team family therapist to steer their way through all these issues, for physicians are singularly unqualified to do this. If for no other reason than the effect good family therapy has on the general quality of life for the whole family, physicians should not attempt to single-handedly manage children with anorexia nervosa.

One of the greatest challenges for the family therapist, in this age of multiple divorces, is to bring the parents around to the view that regardless of history and animosity, they must work together again for the sake of their child. The team must not be coerced into taking sides, even when it is difficult not to. To go along with one parent refusing to "be in the same room" with the other, or insisting that the "new wife" or "new husband" be excluded is to reinforce a family structure and *modus operandi* that will sabotage ordered eating and a calm environment for the child. The doctors must support the family therapists in their effort to be wise and even-handed.

One of the more unique jobs of the family therapists in our clinic is to *check the family's adherence to and understanding of the meal plan.* In other clinics nutritionists or dieticians usually do this job, but over the years, I have found that there is so much emotional content to dietary recommendations that family therapists are better trained to deal with them. We have taught our family therapists the principles of the food plan, they have access to Web-based calorie and fat counters if they need to answer simple food adjustment questions from the parents, and they review the written records families are required to bring to every appointment. If families do not have their recorded food journal (FJ) with them when they come for appointments, they will usually not be seen. Changes in the meal plan, caloric additions, subtractions, and substitutions are done by the doctors, but the family therapists are the "check and balance" on actual compliance. And more importantly, family therapists serve as a sounding board for distress caused by food issues within the family. This is hard work, let me tell you!

## Group therapy

To repeat what we mentioned about group therapy in the chapter on day treatment: "Group" is the one place where the patients can be themselves with no doctors and no parents around. During group therapy the patients interact in a guided peer group, and "group" is where they tell us what is really going on with them.

Although it is very census-dependent at any given time, we try to have as many different homogeneous outpatient groups going as we can. For example: "Young patient AN-R group" (for restrictors under age 14), "older patient AN-R group" (for restrictors from 14 through their junior year in high school), "boys' group" (when census allows this division), "teens with purging or binge-purging group," "seniors group" (kids who are seniors in high school and need to work on independent eating away from home), "college-aged group" (for graduates of the CA-DTU), and so forth.

We have come to feel that peer-guided groups (no therapist present), such as those found at many colleges, can be counter-productive and serve more as competitive "who is or was the sickest" groups than as actual support forums. Don't believe me? Ask the kids.

## Individual therapy

In the treatment of pediatric eating disorders, individual therapy takes a backseat to family therapy and group therapy. In some cases, however, such as a history of trauma, a nonverbal or poorly verbal child, or one with autism or other co-occurring conditions that make a group setting less helpful, we recommend individual therapy.

There is much conflict in the literature about what modes of therapy work best [44]. As a team we try to assign an individual therapist based on our guess of what the best fit will be: Art therapy, play therapy, hypnotherapy [124], drug and alcohol evaluation and treatment, cognitive behavioral therapy, and so on. Pet therapy, something used routinely as adjunct therapy in many children's hospitals these days, is also something we use. We were skeptical that it could play a very significant role until we presented our therapy dog to a 9-year-old boy who would not eat or talk and who was so fearful of the doctors he was curled into a fetal position. When the therapy dog came up to him, his small hand shot out to pet her; within a few minutes the boy had uncurled and would even speak a little as long as the dog was there for him to touch. The therapy dog has worked very well for one of our patients with autism and food phobia as well. For most kids, especially in a group setting, the dog is a source of amusement, an ice breaker for the shy.

## Medication

In medicine we use medication for one major reason: To alleviate suffering. Whether suffering takes the form of physical pain, psychological pain (insomnia, grief, intractable anxiety), or the pain of loss of function is irrelevant. The stigma of "brain disorders" or "mental illness" is still such that taking medication for conditions considered psychological (brain based) is seen as a weakness or character flaw or even as an addiction. During our informational discussion with the parents before beginning any medication we try to normalize the fact that in our branch of medicine, just like all the others, we use the most up-to-date pharmacological interventions available. For extensive details on which medications we currently use and why, please see Dr. Desocio's chapter on Psychopharmacology.

Parents: Keep an open mind! Discuss any reservations you have about medication openly with your doctor and monitor your child carefully for side effects. Surely how well your child does is more important than being able to say "we don't believe in medication."

## Dietician

A word about the obvious absence of a dietician in our outpatient program may be in order here. It is emphatically not because I do not value dieticians. Rather, although I understand that I am nearly alone in this opinion, I feel that the training of a dietician/nutritionist is wasted in the outpatient treatment of anorexia nervosa. Our patients are already world-class experts on food values. Want to know how many grams of fat in a turkey sandwich? How many calories in 8 ounces of orange juice? Just ask a young person with anorexia nervosa. They know all about what they should eat; it's getting them to do it that counts. In our program "Getting them to do it," it is the role of the physician, who has the authority to enforce what is clearly medically indicated.

# 15.5     The outpatient course of illness in anorexia nervosa

## Remission

Most patients are not in complete remission by the time they get to the outpatient clinic. For them *remission* will be the outpatient goal. An occasional child will essentially have reached remission by the time they are discharged from the DTU. For them *consolidation of remission* is the goal.

What is remission?

For intuitive reasons we divide remission into two large categories: Physiological and psychological. It has been our experience that children usually go into physiological remission ahead of psychological remission. But don't despair! This is one of those circumstances in which the physician (and the family) is well advised to rely on "tincture of time." Healing takes time.

*Physiological remission* includes the following:

1. Weight restoration either to their premorbid weight (their weight before they got ill) or to a weight that allows them to resume menstruation (in girls old enough to have periods), have normal hormonal status (girls and boys), and/or to grow.

2. No more restricting, bingeing, or purging, and eating a balanced diet on the meal plan.

3. Back to normal physical activities such as sports or playing (for young children).

*Psychological remission* includes the following:

1. Going back to school and doing well.

2. Interacting with friends and having a normal social life.

3. Having a normal family life.

4. Being able to control symptoms of anxiety such as over-exercising, insomnia , and worry.

5. Acceptance of their bodies, at least enough to have normal age-appropriate relationships.

6. Return of sense of humor and laughter.

7. Ability to ignore any eating disorder thoughts if they arise.

## Resumption of menses

I have picked this particular aspect out of "physiological remission" for reasons that will become obvious. It will, of course, only pertain to girls old enough to have had a period or who hope to get one. I strongly suspect that, bound as menstruation is to normal hormonal functioning, a similar situation exists with boys, at least in respect to testosterone levels (which we know are low in starvation) but there is too little research to support this yet.

The first reason that it matters whether or not a girl regains enough weight to convince her body to resume menstruation is because of her bones. Remember, it doesn't matter how much calcium you ingest as a female, if you don't have estrogen you won't be able to absorb and use it. Giving estrogen (via hormone or birth control pills) does not help, and the window of opportunity to put on new bone growth closes after the mid twenties. That may seem like a long away off to the parents of a young teen, but we have seen many, many patients who looked weight restored, but who never achieved menstruation because neither they nor their parents could accept that she might have to weigh more than she considers acceptable or *more than she ever did before*. A young woman may be diagnosed with an eating disorder when she is seventeen, for example, having been symptomatic usually for at least a year before. She may have been treated but never restored to a weight where her periods could return, and gone off to college, only to later find herself osteopenic at twenty-six or seven, having moved beyond the window of opportunity for bone growth. What a pity!

The second reason resumption of menses matters is psychological. Young girls and women may be deeply ambivalent about getting a period, believing it means they are finally "fat" enough, but in the end most young women want to "be normal" in this respect. Here is one case where I say: "Let's be normal."

But the final reason for focusing on a return of menstruation is, in my view, even more important than the first two. Debra Katzman and co-investigators at the Hospital for Sick Children in Toronto have studied the impact of weight and menstrual functioning on brain structure and function in adolescents and concluded that menstrual recovery may be more important to cognition than even weight recovery. Apparently estrogen enhanced 5HT-IA and 2A receptors are involved in working memory and executive functioning [55]. What does this mean? It means that your child's brain is at risk if she is allowed to hold on to a "socially acceptable weight" even though it means that she never resumes (or achieves) normal menstruation. This is particularly important research to be aware of if your daughter is an athlete and you are told not to worry because "all runners miss their periods" or "no one on the track team, swim team, ski team, dance team, etc. has a period." I don't know about you, but I think the brain is the most important organ in the body: It is who we really are.

# Relapse

It's a tough thing to say, but anorexia nervosa is a chronic condition of remission and exacerbation (relapse) . In our experience, nearly everyone relapses at some time. The trick is to recognize relapse *early* and get the anorexia nervosa back into remission quickly—no harm, no foul. It is not the end of the world when a child relapses unless the disease is allowed to spin out of control and engulf the child emotionally. And boy, can that happen fast! Forewarned is forearmed, and you will be a good judge of your own child if you keep an open mind to the possibility. Parents experience pain and anguish at the thought of relapse—even almost PTSD-like symptoms (post-traumatic stress disorder), which puts them at high danger of "denial." Don't let it catch you unawares, depress you or make you feel hopeless or helpless. You are not helpless, far from it. Just don't sit there hoping it will go away.

If your child shows signs of relapsing such as struggling with meal completion, hiding food, secretly exercising, engaging in tearful discussions about who is eating what, social isolation and (of course) weight loss, stay calm. The intensity of treatment will need to increase for a while, but unless you ignore this and let it go on, you are not "back at square one." Adequate treatment will have supplied some internal resiliency that may not be apparent to the naked eye. When relapse is diagnosed early enough, achieving remission will not take as long as it did the first time, usually not nearly as long. Just don't wait.

# 15.6   Weight gain and body fat redistribution

At no point along the continuum of care at the Kartini Clinic do we discuss a patient's actual weight with them. The doctors establish a weight goal, and they monitor it. If a patient is losing weight, food is added; if they gain weight too rapidly or beyond the established goal weight, food is removed. If they are gaining weight on the minimum calories shown above, we look for bingeing or snacking off the plan. And if they are eating on their meal plan, normally active and not engaged in any eating disordered behaviors and their weight is going up, it is because it needs to. We guessed too low. It happens.

Although we do sometimes get requests from our patients to discuss their weight openly, it is our firm policy never to do so. Once they adjust to this and understand that *there is no way we will make an exception* they are oddly comforted. They have transferred the responsibility and the anxiety about their weight to our shoulders. Do any of our patients ever weigh themselves? Of course. And when they do, they get upset. We work through why this was a bad idea for them and caused them needless pain. Besides, invariably the weight on the scale in the gym or the one they found under their parents' bed, is higher than the one we recorded in the office where they were weighed without clothes and after a void. Eventually even oppositional (usually older) patients finally agree it is counterproductive for them to follow their own weight numbers.

One of the more distressing things about weight gain following semi-starvation is the distribution of fat that follows. We confront this issue directly in the outpatient clinic; there is no point trying to hide from the elephant in the room: The human body stores initial weight gain around the face and stomach. Some children may appear to be "chubby" to their parents once they reach their weight goal. Of course they are not "chubby," but at this point it is essential to continue the frank discussion (begun in the DTU) about *weight redistribution.* We do not know why it happens or understand the mechanism involved, but we have consistently observed that the extra weight gained at first around the face and stomach will redistribute over time. How soon? Boy, would I be popular if I could accurately predict that! It usually takes several months to happen, but when it does, it is fairly sudden and rather dramatic. In the outpatient clinic I sometimes think a child has lost weight, but when I check their chart, I see that this is not so; the puffiness and extra fat has merely "left the face" with the tummy to follow. Really. The kids are very pleased, the parents are relieved, and the doctors are happy, too.

One last word about measuring weight in any outpatient setting, whether you are a doctor, a nurse or a parent: Be skeptical, be wise. It is easy to fool a doctor, nurse, or parent about weight (just ask the kids), so always use the same scale every time. If you are far away from the same scale, don't weigh the child at all. Unnecessary weigh-ins cause anxiety. We weigh only because we have to and it is the trend we are looking for. Remember, when weight restoring a child, two steps forward and one step back is not acceptable. The curve must always be up. Weight gain may not be real (and can be faked), but weight loss is always real.

Weigh the patient or your child with their back to the scales, get rid of mirrors in the weighing area, weigh in a gown or the same basic set of underwear each time, some light article of clothing that does not allow them to hide weights. Weigh only after a void (urination), check the child physically for weights, and check the urine specific gravity (if you are a medical provider) for water loading. There are tricks to making your weight look like it's increased, all of which the kids taught us. We have had more than one patient endanger their toes from weights falling out from under their arms or vaginal area. Nice try.

## 15.7   Ideal body weight

Establishing or determining ideal body weight has been extensively discussed in the chapter on inpatient stabilization. Below I include a few outpatient examples of real children facing the issue of their own return to a goal weight.

**Case 1:** "Susie" represents the case of a 17-year-old girl who has had restricting anorexia nervosa for three years. Her menarche (first menstruation) had occurred at 12 years of age, and her periods were regular until they ceased at about age 14. She received therapy from a psychologist for the first two years of her illness, but by the time she came to our attention, she was 16 years old, weighed 100 pounds, and was bradycardic (low heart rate) and amenorrheic (no longer menstruating). She gained weight in the hospital and in the day treatment unit and was discharged to outpatient care weighing 121.5 pounds. She is 65 inches tall and weighed 135 pounds before she got sick, at age 14. Her bone density study, done in the hospital, showed that she had severe osteopenia (weak bones) so her parents were interested in her resuming normal menstrual functioning even though she "didn't care about her period," she just "didn't want to be fat again." At 122 pounds she resumed bleeding, and her hormone level was in the lowest range possible for resuming menstruation so she did not want to "gain even one more ounce." That seemed fair, but as time went on, even though she followed her food plan of 2,150 kcals/day to the letter and returned to her cheerleading activities, she continued to gain weight. She discovered that to keep her weight below 125 pounds (the "ideal weight" she had read about online using the formula of 100 pounds for 5 feet and 5 pounds for each additional inch) she needed to practice "restrained eating" and eat only about 1,800 kcals/day. Not only was it hard to convince Susie that she would need to take in adequate calories to sustain her energy output, but Susie's mother was also convinced that it "wasn't fair," because there were girls who were Susie's height and thinner than she was who were "perfectly healthy." This was a set-up for deep unhappiness for Susie since neither she nor her mother (who also had many weight concerns of her own) were able to accept that Susie's body was not designed to function at this very lean weight she yearned for and that her body would try to return to her former plateau.

**Discussion:** As hard as it is to tell patients and their families what they don't want to hear, Susie was apparently not genetically programmed to function at a weight this low (125 pounds) and would need to engage in eating-disordered behaviors to remain there. If she were to do this, she could never get out of the trap of constantly supervising her weight and worrying about it—not to mention that a low level of restricting would set her up for bingeing. In our clinic this is the kind of situation that will need extensive family work to help Susie's mother accept the biology involved. Likely, Susie will also need individual therapy to be able to gradually accept the wisdom of her own body and to like herself the way she is. Treating physicians will need to have a good understanding of these issues or they can make them worse.

**Case 2:** "Alli" is the case of a 16-year-old girl who was diagnosed with restricting anorexia nervosa when she was 14 and

had "had her illness for less than a year by that age." The most
Alli had ever weighed (around age 14) was 120 pounds. She is
tall (67.5 inches) and comes from a family of very active, long,
lean people on both sides. She did not require hospitalization, but
went straight to the day treatment unit and was then followed
in the outpatient clinic. She gained weight slowly from a low of
108 pounds to a "high" of 127 pounds. At that point her periods,
while present, were very irregular. A quick calculation showed that
her BMI at 127 pounds was 19.5 (probably too low for her) and
that a weight of 130 pounds would yield a BMI of 20 (probably
more supportive of normal, regular, ovulatory menses) and she
would still be quite slender. These numbers were shared with Alli's
mother, who was distressed and puzzled since 127–130 pounds was
"more than Alli had ever weighed." Once Alli's weight went up her
periods normalized. And at 130 lbs and five feet seven and a half,
she was still slender with a BMI of 20.

**Discussion:** Alli is now 16, and was eventually able to accept
her "new normal" weight. It was helpful to be able to share
with both Alli and her Mom research by Neville Golden and
colleagues showing that many patients need to weigh *more* to
resume menstruation than they before they got ill [37].

**Case 3:** "Bob" is a 17-year-old boy who was diagnosed with restricting anorexia nervosa accompanied by episodes of bingeing not
followed by vomiting, but rather by intense bouts of compensatory
exercising. He was 6 feet, 2 inches tall and weighed 210 pounds
before he got ill and a year later weighed 159 pounds. Because he
was weak and bradycardic (low heart rate), he was admitted to
the hospital and, once stabilized, transferred to the DTU. A bone
density study showed him to have osteoporosis and his testosterone
level was quite low. Bob had noticed a decrease in libido. By
the time his weight was up to 190 pounds, his testosterone level

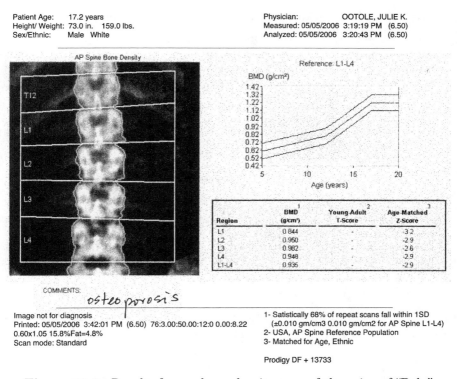

**Figure 15.2:** Results from a bone density scan of the spine of "Bob."

had risen to normal and his energy had returned to normal. His low temperature had resolved, and his heart rate had gone from a resting average rate in the low 40s (and 30s at night) to the 60-70s. He had been eating 3,700 kcals/day to support this level of restoration, but at this point the doctors began "dialing back" on his calories to approach a more average intake of 3,000 kcals/day since his physiologic parameters had normalized.

**Discussion:** We knew Bob was no longer bingeing because his parents kept an "exact book" on his intake, with his cooperation; it had not been our intention to return him to his former weight of 210 pounds, if we could avoid it, because this would put him above the 95th percentile (the same as his height). Not having a marker for biological normalcy in boys like we do in girls (menstruation), we are more in the dark about what weight to consider "ideal" in a boy, especially a growing boy, as the next case illustrates. This being the case, we try to normalize those biologic parameters that we can measure such as heart rate, hormone levels, orthostatic vitals, and temperature. We consider that a boy will likely be "weight restored" when these things are normal and when his energy and mood are again normal, provided he is not still engaging in eating disordered behaviors. If Bob had needed to exercise compulsively to stay at 190 pounds or had hidden or skipped food, this would likely not be his "ideal body weight " and we would have to accept the higher weight.

**Case 4:** "Myron" represents a 10-year-old boy diagnosed with early-onset anorexia nervosa, restricting subtype. His symptoms probably began at about age eight. Looking at the growth curve his pediatrician forwarded to us, we saw that he begin to fall off his normal growth curve before age nine, moving from the 50th percentile to the 25th percentile by nine and now being below the 5th percentile at age 10. His height growth flattened out from the 50th percentile to the 25th percentile. His weight was 53 pounds on admission to the hospital, where we were able—despite his intense anxiety—to move him back up to 63 pounds (his highest weight ever recorded). As his weight began to move up from there toward 70 pounds (the 50 percentile for a 10-year-old boy), his face rounded out (causing some consternation in the parents), but at that point Myron began to grow.

**Discussion:** Myron will clearly have to be returned to a weight higher than he has ever experienced before because he is growing and because his normal growth had been stunted. Returning him to the 50th percentile seemed a logical place to start; he was Tanner I (prepubertal) at the outset, so measurements of testosterone seem unlikely to be very helpful. On the other hand, his admission low heart rate disappeared with weight restoration, his temperature normalized and—best of all—he began to grow, allaying his father's concern that we were going to "make him chubby." (See figures 15.3 and 15.4.)

## 15.8　Impediments to healing a child

There are many circumstances which can present impediments to a child's healing from anorexia nervosa. Some are intuitive, some unexpected. All require facing head on. I am going to start out with the least intuitive and most difficult one to talk frankly about:

### Other affected family members

Anorexia nervosa has a strong genetic component to it, as we discussed in the chapter on genetics. One of the implications of this is that it is quite common to find more than one affected family member in an extended family. We take careful histories from the beginning of our relationship with the family and add to them as more family members "come forward" with their own medical and mental health histories. It is not uncommon for one (or both) of the parents to also be affected or to have a history of an eating disorder "in the past." It is not always the same eating disorder: A girl with anorexia nervosa may have a sister with bulimia nervosa, a grandfather with selective eating, and a female cousin who had to see the doctor many times for "not having periods."

　　Families who carry whatever gene(s) are involved in this vulnerability to anorexia nervosa also commonly inherit a tendency toward perfectionism and anxiety disorders (panic attacks, pho-

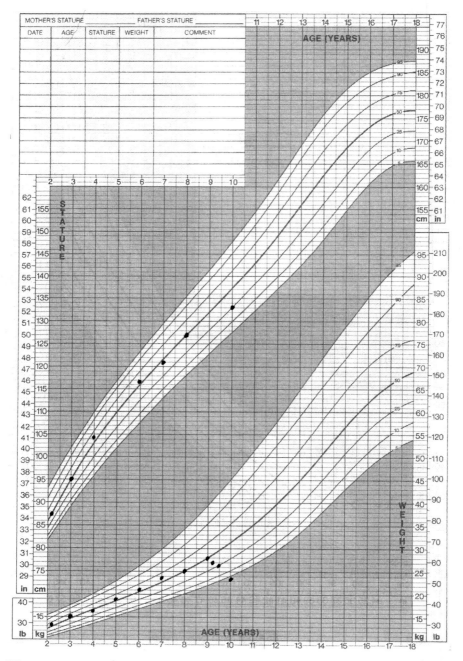

**Figure 15.3:** Height and weight growth chart on "Myron" looking back from age 10.

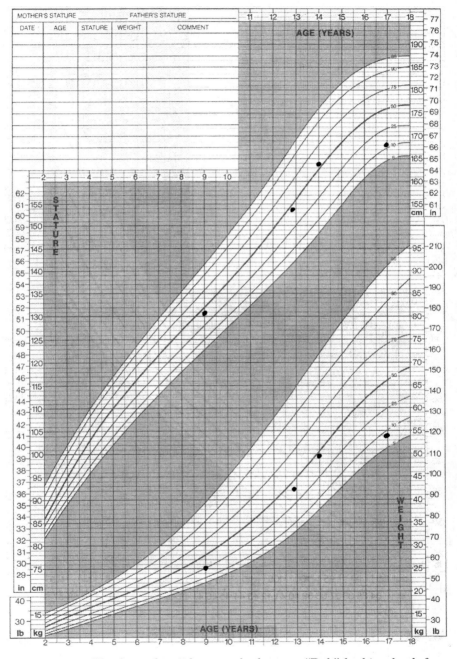

**Figure 15.4:** Height and weight growth chart on "Bob" looking back from age 17.

bias, generalized anxiety disorder, obsessive-compulsive disorder or traits, social phobia [128] [114] [57] [66] [5]). What this will mean in practice is that other family members besides just the patient who has been brought to us may have significant anxiety about weight when required by our family-based treatment to prepare and eat family meals. It is not uncommon for the also affected family member to be the mother, because anorexia and bulimia are more common in women, and it is not uncommon for a mother who brought her child to us for treatment to begin herself to have conflicted feelings about food and weight as her child's treatment progresses. This can and will interfere with her child's treatment, unless addressed compassionately but promptly.

So let's stick with this hypothetical mother (it could of course have been the father) whose own eating issues have been triggered by her daughter's treatment. How could she actually "interfere with treatment?"

What we commonly see is that once an affected parent's own fears have been aroused, and their own body image issues re-kindled, they may be unable to enforce the meal plan or accept necessary weight gain in their child. They may actually uncon-sciously slip into coalition with their child's eating disorder and begin to allow him or her to skip meals or add-ons, concealing this from the team so he/she "won't get into trouble." In its most tragic and destructive form, the affected parent, out of fear and anxiety, confusion and ambivalence, actually agrees with their child that "the team has made him/her gain too much weight" and that he/she "should be allowed to lose at least a little weight." You can imagine what that means for treatment.

Now I know I am on shaky ground here with those who might begin to fear that I am blaming the parent just described or that I am somehow saying that a parent who has ever had an eating disorder themselves cannot care for their own eating disordered child. I am saying nothing of the kind. I am merely saying that eating disorders run in families and we must gently but firmly face this fact. Where we see other family members whose issues have been triggered by family-based treatment, we must find help for them as well and not hesitate to speak honestly.

We once had a 20-year-old patient whose parents had removed her against medical advice from treatment several times, who came to us the final time as a wasted skeleton weighing 64 pounds at 65 inches tall. Her parents pleaded with us to help her this one last time. Her teeth were rotten from vomiting, her bones brittle from eight years of inadequate weight. With a huge amount of effort in the hospital and DTU our team brought her weight up slowly to 120 pounds. She was beautiful, and she actually had a period, the first in many, many years. She got a scholarship to college; she was smart, funny and talented. Because she did not stay at this weight long enough for the above-referenced weight redistribution to take place, her face and stomach were a little rounded. Incredibly, it was at this point that the father (who had an eating disorder himself) began to tell her that we had made her fat; her mother subsequently withdrew her from treatment, saying she "agreed with her daughter that she should lose some weight." At home her weight quickly went down into the 50-60 lb range. We were heart broken.

Whenever a family history reveals that a first-degree relative (parent, sibling) who lives with the child we are treating also has an eating disorder, it is important to address this directly but sympathetically. It has been our experience that if the affected family member does not get treatment for their own eating disorder, the child we are treating will not get well. They will trigger one another constantly. Fortunately parents will occasionally do things

for the sake of their child (e.g. seek treatment) that they would
not do for their own sake.

## Misguided medical providers

As a medical provider and because doctors are famously defensive of
one another, I write this section reluctantly. I hope that physicians
and other practitioners who treat children may learn from the
mistakes of those who have gone before them. What follows is a
list of common problems that either delay effective treatment or
make complete restoration impossible or unlikely. I cannot tell you
how often a family tells us that the doctor they trust and admire
falsely consoled them about their child' weight loss until it was
too late for them to be re-fed outside the hospital.

**Ignoring failure to thrive:** Starting with the worst, this is
perhaps more a doctor's failure to look at their own office growth
chart than anything else. I have had many children referred
to me, boys and girls, who have clearly failed to thrive, whose
growth charts show them to have dropped in weight across several
percentiles over the course of some years, followed by a flattening of
the growth curve for height. Whether or not this growth stunting
is reversible depends on how long it has been allowed to go on and
what Tanner stage (SMR) the patient has achieved by the time it is
diagnosed. I have had more than one boy with a growth curve like
this who, when bone age X-rays were taken, was discovered to have
no further growth potential. In other words, their growth had been
permanently stunted. Usually the parents are so stunned by this
bad news and so self-blaming that they do not blame the physician
particularly; however, I think all pediatric providers would agree
that this represents a severe failure of good care. Please do not let

this happen to your child. Either make your doctor listen to your concerns or find one who will (see figures 15.3 and 15.4).

**Praising weight loss when it is not clear on what basis this has been achieved:** Our clinic is full of angry parents who report that either their doctor or their child's coach or health teacher told their eating-disordered child, "Good for you, you are exercising and cutting out all fats!" Weight loss might be a good thing for certain people, but it behooves a person, especially one in a position of authority or credibility, to know whereof he or she speaks before they say anything.

**Giving an unrealistic weight goal to a child who has an eating disorder:** I can't tell you how often a patient tells me, "But my pediatrician (or my coach or my health teacher or my aunt who is a nurse...) says I should weigh 120 pounds because I'm five four," when that *particular* child has no periods and is weak at that weight. Pronouncements about where a child's weight should be are best left to those who know how to do it. Once the words are out: "I think you should weigh..." They are almost impossible to retract.

## Misguided mental health providers

Perhaps because we are a medically oriented clinic we get fewer misguided comments from our mental health colleagues than from our physician colleagues, but when we do, they are major! Following are a few of the unfortunate comments we have heard:

- You can't have anorexia nervosa because you are not thin enough.

- Everybody purges occasionally.

- Your parents caused this.

- The eating disorder is just an expression of other, non-food-related struggles, which we need to get to the bottom of.

- Having an eating disorder means you have been sexually abused, whether you can remember it or not.

- Your son's eating disorder means he is gay.

- You have a sugar allergy/addiction, and that is causing all your eating problems.

- You are regurgitating your mother. Find out why.

- Unless you "buy into" your treatment, it can't help.

- Your parents need to "butt out" of your meal plans and food.

## Family pressure to "be normal"

This is an interesting human problem, one I think all parents can relate to. We want our children to be happy; we want them to be *normal*. Now, I am not saying that eating-disordered patients are not normal; in every way that does not relate to their eating disorder and to food, they usually are normal, very fine kids. But as a child with dwarfism is not "normal" when it comes to height and one with cerebral palsy is not "normal" when it comes to ambulation, so children with anorexia nervosa and its variants are not "normal" when it comes to food. People with eating disorders cannot self-regulate around food. Some people are eventually able to relate normally to food after treatment, though usually not for some time. It has been my experience that some pediatric patients are not "normal" about food for years. Pressure to "be normal" or to "eat like everyone else," is unrealistic, unfair, counterproductive, and can increases anxiety. If a child with anorexia nervosa is able to eat his or her required meal plan consisting of real food with adequate heart-healthy fats, *that is absolutely a home run* and should be seen as such.

For years I taught a nutrition group to parents and their children with anorexia nervosa. One of the most common questions was, "When can my child eat off the plan? I mean, can she have birthday cake?" I would look at the child and say, "Do you want birthday cake?" Almost all the "restrictors" would vehemently shake their heads "No!" and the parents would be nonplussed: "But you used to love birthday cake!" Well, that's exactly the point: If they didn't love it, they wouldn't be afraid to have it around. Some of the "purgers" would say that they wanted the cake, but when they realized that they would not be allowed to restrict food from their meals if they did eat the cake and therefore could not "get rid of it," they did not want it either. Many children have told me that they are afraid that if they eat one piece of cake, they won't be able to stop, or that they would feel so guilty, they would have to exercise off what they ate as quickly as possible or else restrict food from their meal plan. At the very least such normal snacking would cause them anxiety, and the whole point of ordered eating is *to reduce anxiety.* Attempts to insist that a child "eating normally" is the only acceptable treatment outcome are, in my opinion, misguided.

## Health class at school

We get four or five case reports a year about anorexia nervosa starting "after health class at school." Often this is in the setting of a pitch by the health teacher for students to learn to "cut the fats out of their diet," "increase their physical activity," and monitor their weight and body fat. Sometimes the kids have even been weighed in the class or have had their skinfold thickness measured. This is very triggering talk for eating disordered kids, but imagine how humiliating this experience would be for overweight kids. Almost no one who is overweight responds to public humiliation by improving their diet. Yet, self-image in a child can be dramatically worsened. Young people with (incipient) anorexia nervosa attending a health class where the emphasis is how fat everyone is today may also respond differently than the teacher intended. Weight control advice that other children may take in stride, ignore, or use to transiently change their health practices, supercharges an eating-disordered or anxious child's determination to "become more perfect." Their secret fear that they are "too big," "not fit enough," or "eating all the wrong things" receives validation in the form of the authority of the health teacher. Be careful, be very, very careful how you handle children and their perceptions of their own growing bodies.

I disagree strongly with children being weighed or having their fat measured in any public setting. I understand that it is done to try to solve the problem of obesity, but to my knowledge such humiliation has never made a fat kid thinner. Our current practice at the Kartini Clinic is to excuse eating-disordered patients from health class, or at least those aspects of health class that have to do with food, diet, fat, or eating disorders. Our young patients consistently report health class discussions about eating disorders to be intensely triggering: Pictures of starved persons with anorexia not only don't repulse them, but actually make them jealous (remember, it's a brain disorder). Eating disordered children cannot be dissuaded from their behaviors by being shown how starvation affects the body. This is like showing depressed patients pictures of weeping family members whose lives have been worsened by the patient's mental illness. It's counterproductive and deeply flawed.

Eating-disordered patients do, however, like all other children, need to learn about safe sex, proper immunization, seat belts, car safety, and so on, and should participate in those sections of a health class. However, the very last thing they should ever do is to speak to the class about eating disorders as a resident expert (see "No Professional Anorexics" below).

## Sports pressure

Athletic ability and interest in physical activity seems to run in families; those children who are very athletic often have at least one parent who is likewise interested in sports. There is also a widespread belief that sports protect adolescents from the influence of drugs and alcohol and the pervasive curse of obesity [22]. With all this good press, how can we criticize athletics? I do not criticize athletics, as such, as long as we do not forget the whole child. A child should have an integrated social, academic, spiritual, and family life as well as their body-centered life. If an averagely athletic child becomes a committed, fanatic exerciser in the course of their eating disorder, this should obviously not be encouraged *regardless of the success he or she garners from it.*

Occasionally a problem of a different sort will arise: Once the eating-disordered thoughts are under control, the child may lose interest in sports, severely disappointing sports-minded parents who then may put pressure on them to continue with the basketball team, the wrestling team, or the track team. When that doesn't work, they may put pressure on the eating-disorder team to insist that the child be returned to his or her former "healthy activity." The coach, who has a lot of credibility with young people, may not understand the approach of the treatment team or may even actively oppose it. The patient may have an athletic scholarship, he or she may report deriving their "self-esteem" solely from his or her sports ability. . . it makes for a nightmare. The only recourse is to discuss these issues openly from the beginning and, where possible, make the coach a team member.

## 15.9   No professional anorexics

A final word needs to be said on the subject of what we call "professional anorexics." Once more I am highly aware that not everyone will agree with me on this subject. We must be clear about our treatment goals for our children: We want them to be the best, most accomplished, and happiest person they can be. The last thing we want is for them to so identify with their illness that they write all their term papers on eating disorders, write their college essay on "how I overcame anorexia," and go on to become nutritionists or doctors specializing in this subject. I would rather they were astronauts, writers, mothers, senators, fathers. . . anything but "professional anorexics." Leave the disease behind! Leave it behind!

Sadly, we encounter patients, usually older ones, whose illness (from which they may have "recovered") has become the focus of their life and their self-vision. Their involvement in anorexia nervosa has become total. The ego syntonic nature of their relationship to their illness means they can never leave it behind them.

This is how we advise parents: Please do not have your child give conferences and talks about eating disorders, mentor others at school, or become the "go-to guy" for others on the subject, for although it is understandable that they might feel they have something to offer, let's go back to the early treatise on anorexia nervosa by Richard Morton, from in the late 1600s and never forget that "at first it flatters and deceives the patient." Identification with the illness will lead the child away from healing. Let them be treated early and adequately and go forth, healed, to be a person who has an illness but who is not that illness, who has experienced the pain but who has moved beyond that. In short, let them be like every other child.

## Clinical pearls

- The Meal Plan is an anxiety-reduction tool.

- The Meal Plan ensures weight restoration in the beginning but ensures a cap on weight gain in the end.

- Following an episode of semi-starvation, unwanted overeating is common.

- Early weight gain is commonly seen in the face and stomach: This will redistribute.

- Eating-disordered children need to return to school.

- *Parents* are responsible for feeding their children.

- Do not tolerate inadequate weight restoration, continued bone loss, or amenorrhea.

- Do not engage in inadequate treatment.

- Relapse is a normal part of the natural history of the disease and does not necessarily represent a failure of treatment. Keep going!

# 16 Food Phobia

This chapter will discuss what is known about the diagnosis and treatment of the eating disorder we know as "food phobia." It will present our experience with food phobia at the Kartini Clinic and the evolution of our treatment protocols towards an increasingly family-based experience. I will discuss the use of medication and the introduction of food. Finally, I will present two case histories from either end of the pediatric eating disorder spectrum followed by a discussion of treatment options.

I have devoted a separate chapter to food phobia in this book because so little is understood about it in the community of pediatric mental or medical health providers and because treatment has proven very difficult for families to find. As with other pediatric eating disorders described so far, there is a spectrum of severity of illness, with some cases resolving spontaneously, others remitting with relatively brief psychological interventions and still others lasting long enough to severely impact the child's health or even cause death. The older adolescent presented below underscores how dangerous this condition can be if it goes unrecognized and untreated.

Food phobia is described by some authors as "functional dysphagia." a term I prefer not to use because of the historic use of the word "functional" when denying a biological substrate to a given behavior, and also because this condition does not always involve a fear of swallowing as such, but may instead involve a fear of vomiting, suffocating or abdominal pain.

Because typically only those cases which have been refractory to outpatient intervention are referred to the Kartini Clinic, we have primarily treated these patients in an inpatient setting, using neuroleptic medication, nasogastric feeds and a multi-disciplinary approach to psychological recovery. Using the inpatient protocol we developed we have been able to achieve good resolution of symptoms in all cases and a return to normal eating. More recently we have applied the principles of "family-based" treatment to our protocol as will be described below.

## 16.1 Definition

Food phobia of childhood, primarily reported in pre- or early pubertal children, was first described using this term by Bryan Lask (pediatric psychiatrist) and Rachel Bryant-Waugh (clinical psychologist) in the early 1990s as a result of their work at Great Ormond Street Children's Hospital in London [68]. Apart from a scattered few articles on children with a specific phobia involving food, such as the article by Mathew Knock of Yale University in 2002 [87] and another by Singer *et al.* in 1992 [111], food phobia has not been much discussed in the American pediatric literature except under the general term "dysphagia" where it is likely to come to the attention primarily of pediatric gastroenterologists and otolaryngologists. In the adult literature it is sometimes referred to as "choking phobia."

More recently Dr. Lask has chosen to refer to this condition as "functional dysphagia," although, as mentioned, at the Kartini Clinic we prefer the more intuitive "food phobia." In our experience, pediatricians report being at a loss to treat this challenging diagnosis. In fact, the single patient reported in the Knock article was four years old and had been refusing to eat solid food since he was seven months old! We are grateful to Drs. Lask and Bryant-Waugh for calling our attention to this condition. The grateful parents whose children we have successfully treated owe them a debt as well.

Food phobia, then, is the sudden onset of food refusal and may extend to refusal to swallow anything, even the patient's own saliva. Young patients with this condition may easily become undernourished and dehydrated and when the condition has become chronic it is usually because a parent has figured out how to keep their child alive on drinks and semi-solid mixtures or because a desperate practitioner has inserted a gastrostomy tube (G-tube) directly into the stomach through the skin. Children with food phobia ate normally and developed normally prior to the onset of their illness. This is an important point to distinguish it from the various eating and swallowing difficulties of many developmentally delayed children.

The "reason" children with food phobia give for their food refusal is often a fear of choking or a fear of vomiting and/or germ contamination leading to illness; they may report food and water getting "stuck" in their throat or they may simply refuse to talk about why they won't eat or drink. In our experience, onset is usually abrupt; the child is young; there is a family history of anxiety disorders, and the child does not have anorexia nervosa (AN) or bulimia nervosa (BN). There is none of the body dysmorphism or "fat fears" associated with those other diagnoses (AN and BN). The onset of the illness may be preceded by a choking episode, either experienced or witnessed, or even experienced vicariously as when an adult described another child's death by choking. Efforts on the part of the parents to induce their child to eat by bribing, cajoling, threatening, pleading, or rewarding are typically to no avail.

A word about age of onset and prevalence: Because of the relative rarity of this condition and the lack of attention it has received in the pediatric literature, we have no real idea what the prevalence/incidence or age of onset is. It has been our over-whelming experience that patients with food phobia are young (less than thirteen years old), but as we recently successfully treated a very ill 18-year-old, we have to ask ourselves whether or not this perception is an artifact of our being pediatric providers. Are there a lot of older children and even adults with this condition who are simply not referred to us? Is this condition related to the older (adult) literature on so-called "globus hystericus?" How rare is food phobia really? We simply do not know.

## 16.2   Clinical conundrum

After I saw my very first patient with what I now know was food phobia (whom I was unable to help) I was determined to work out a successful treatment protocol. From the beginning it seemed clear that no amount of talking would "convince" a terrified child that he or she was in no danger of choking to death if he or she allowed solid food in his or her mouth. As with anorexia ner-vosa, the SSRIs (selective serotonin reuptake inhibitors), although excellent drugs for anxiety disorders in general, did not seem of much benefit and in any case seemed likely to take too long to work. Most of the children we saw had already undergone some degree of behavioral treatment/desensitization without success. Basically, we were being referred children for whom all of the usual treatment approaches (speech therapy, occupational therapy, behavioral interventions, desensitization) had failed.

## 16.3　Use of medication

Having had good experience with the use of neuroleptics (specifically olanzapine ) in the treatment of refractory childhood-onset anorexia nervosa, we decided to try this class of medication in those with food phobia. The fear of swallowing seemed as delusional as the fear of getting fat and as fixed, so we began with small doses of olanzapine. In short order we discovered that young children required a dose of 7.5 mg/day of olanzepine to begin to respond with any significant reduction in their anxiety. Of course, we conferred from the first with the parents and let them know what we were planning. We discussed the advantages, disadvantages and side-effect profiles of this class of drugs and we advised them that treatment was likely to take weeks. We also added that at first we would not even be talking about food, much less requiring the child to eat it.

## 16.4　Naso-gastric feeds

Once the patient was admitted to the hospital, we placed a naso-gastric tube and started replacement calories as needed to gain any lost weight, along with 2.5 mg of olanzepine at bedtime. The NG tube allowed us all to relax, knowing that the child was getting all the calories, vitamins and fluids that he or she would require to begin to reverse any malnutrition/weight loss. By using the nasogastric route, it was also not necessary for the patient to swallow medication or receive it by injection. No food was introduced until we felt that the child had been adequately re-fed since we knew from experience that the brain could not be malnourished in order for us to have a chance at re-programming it. Parents were encouraged to stay with their child and play games. It would be crucial to gain the confidence of the child, to assure them that they were not going to be punished nor force fed. Timing (and tincture of time!) turned out to be everything.

## 16.5 Waiting... and waiting

At this point we waited for anxiety to abate, the child's anxiety as well as the parents'. I am making this sound easy, but it was not. Food Phobia is among the most difficult things we treat. Some patients we saw were so traumatized by their fears that they would not allow a glass of water or a toothbrush to come near their lips. It was frightening to see a young person so determined never to eat or drink again. We needed all the mutual support of a multi-disciplinary team to keep our own faith in the power of the brain to heal. Some patients would not swallow their own saliva but spit it into a cup they kept at their side. However, it turned out that once the brain was re-fed and the olanzapine had been at a therapeutic level (7.5 mg/day) for a few days, this symptom was the first to abate.

Children with food phobia seem to actually like food, they want to eat, to please their parents, and to get out of the hospital. They do not seem to be trying to lose weight. Their biological drive to eat is not extinguished, only overwhelmed by fear that they will choke or vomit. We are therefore very strict about not offering any food for the first week or so in order to build up a "head of steam" of desire to eat; the biological urge to reward oneself with delicious food is our friend. Then, when "all the stars are aligned" as described above, we start to introduce food.

One of the things we noticed during the waiting period was that the kids often talked a lot about food. They frequently declared they were "ready to eat" and were "going to eat everything" long before they were actually able to do so. Because of this, parents were occasionally upset that we would not immediately begin introducing food. At these times we have found it necessary to ask parents for short-term patience in order to achieve long-term success. Quite a bit of time was spent explaining to parents of our young patients that we might eventually need to resort to behavioral incentives to get over the hump of eating food consistently.

## 16.6   Introducing food: Bite, chew, swallow

Unless the child was very young (say, three years old) we tried not to start introducing solids using soft foods since kids can get stuck there. Sometimes the anxiety had abated enough with the neuroleptic that as soon as we offered food the child was able to eat, each day graduating to more food. But usually it was not quite so simple and we needed to ask the parents to leave in order to give the child a strong incentive to begin to "bite, chew, swallow." When these behavioral incentives were necessary, if the child was able to eat all of breakfast the parent would be allowed to stay with them, otherwise the parents had to leave until lunchtime, at which point the child would have another chance at eating. If the child was then able to eat lunch, their parents could stay, but if not, parents would leave until dinnertime, and so forth. This phase of behavioral reinforcement was almost always the most painful for families and for us.

Our goal was for each child to be able to eat 100% of food offered. Once they were able to eat everything offered, they were transferred to the DTU for a week or two to consolidate eating in a social environment.

**Adding family-based interventions:** Our current protocol is somewhat different from that described above. In 2009 Laura Collins (author of *Eating With Your Anorexic* and founder of the FEAST website for the parents of children with eating disorders) challenged me to incorporate more family-based treatment principles into everything we did. I thought about it. Honestly, I was afraid to tinker with our 100% success rate in treating food phobia, but I had to ask myself: Could we shorten treatment if we took the majority of treatment out of the hospital? Could we teach parents to do what our hospital nurses had always done before? Could we make it less traumatic, less costly? Could we dispense with most or all of the behavioral (dis)incentives? Could parents function less as bystanders and more as treatment providers?

In 2009 we admitted our first patients under our new treatment protocol. It called for the child to be admitted to the hospital for placement of a nasogastric (NG) tube, initial labs, introduction of neuroleptic medication, and treatment of any emergent re-feeding issues. Once this was done, the nurses then would teach parents how to give tube feeds at home (or in the Ronald McDonald House for those families from far away) and discharge them to our day treatment unit (DTU). For most kids this would mean a hospital stay of two days instead of many weeks.

Once in the DTU, the treatment plan was essentially as described earlier, only in a less restrictive, more family-friendly setting: The child's dose of olanzapine was gradually increased to

7.5 mg at bedtime, no food was offered, play and fun with staff and other patients was introduced while we waited. We learned to listen better to parental input about their child's individual food preferences. Once the doctors and therapists felt it had a chance to succeed, we would begin to introduce food.

Introducing food: That's the scary part. That's the best part. To watch a child begin to trust, to close their eyes and begin to let their hunger lead them where you want them to go, to laugh with you and glow when you praise them, there are no words for how rewarding this is. After food had been reintroduced by the doctors, therapists and other special staff members took over. A parent joined us in the re-feeding once their child had swallowed their first bites of food. Slowly—or quickly, if tolerated—food intake was advanced and the tube removed. Once we achieved "bite, chew, swallow," and our staff felt there were no related anxiety issues to address, the child was discharged home on a tapering dose of olanzapine.

**Relapse:** I am commonly asked how often symptoms recur once a child with food phobia has been released from treatment and allowed to go home and back to their pediatrician.

To date, we have not seen symptoms recur in a completely treated patient. One successfully treated six year old boy, who had been tapered off his olanzapine, was given an intranasal flu vaccination by his pediatrician back home; it caused him to choke and gag. This caused an increase in his anxiety and the onset of poor eating; we simply put him back on the medication (olanzepine) for two weeks and his anxiety subsided. Our last contact with his family had him eating, playing and going to school normally, off all medication.

Three patients who were removed by their parents from our program before their treatment was completed experienced incomplete resolution of their symptoms. However, to the date of this writing, to our knowledge, no one who has completed treatment has reported a recurrence of their symptoms. Once extinguished, food phobia seems to be gone for good. In this respect it is quite unlike other childhood eating disorders such as AN or BN, in our experience.

## 16.7　Food phobia case histories

**Five-year-old boy treated using our inpatient protocol:** T.H. was a five year old male from a southern state who presented with a two month history of food refusal. Three weeks prior to the onset of his problem, T.H.'s father told us that his son had awakened in a panic worrying that he had "swallowed a marble." T.H. was able to be reassured by his father and his pediatrician, but then during a subsequent family dinner, gagged on a mouthful of chicken and potatoes. For several days he insisted that he had a chicken bone stuck in his throat. He developed a fever and was taken to the ER where a neck X-ray was read as normal. T.H. continued to refuse all solid food and was subsequently "kept alive" on milk.

T.H. was evaluated by a local psychologist who suggested that the family stop feeding him milk and begin restricting his TV time until he "complied" with eating normally. Force-feeding was attempted and failed. The parents were told they were perpetuating his refusal by allowing him to drink milk.

At the Kartini Clinic T.H. weighed 35 pounds (87.5% of his pre-morbid weight of 40 pounds). Treatment was explained to his father who stayed with him in the hospital where we inserted a nasogastric tube for nutritional stabilization. Olanzapine was begun at 2.5 mg/day and titrated up to 7.5 mg/day over about 8-9 days. After this time, once he was comfortable that the staff liked him and was not going to punish him or "take his TV time away," the doctors began to feed him bananas and yogurt. The first bites were the hardest and he needed a lot of repeated reassurance that the "doctors would never ever let him choke and that he was completely safe in the hospital with us." After two and a half weeks in hospital, once he was able to swallow even a little food, he was transferred to our DTU and was discharged home eating normally after 3 days on a tapering schedule of olanzepine.

If we were to treat a child like T.H. today, we would discharge him directly to the DTU once his nasogastric tube was secured and his father taught to use it. Once able to achieve that "first swallow" we would then have had his father help us to re-feed him in the less restrictive environment of the DTU.

**18-year-old male:** J.B. was an 18-year-old male with a history of anxiety and depression who presented to a small town urgent care facility complaining of an acute episode of "breathlessness" following meals. He was diagnosed there with asthma and a "throat infection." Shortly after this visit he stopped eating all solids complaining of severe sore throat, nausea, fear of vomiting, and abdominal pain. He underwent numerous medical and surgical evaluations: Laboratory testing, imaging (MRI and CT), surgical and gastrointestinal consults, but as J.B.'s symptoms progressed, he became unable to tolerate any fluids including his own saliva.

J.B. had weighed 270 lbs before he got ill and began to rapidly lose weight. He complained that any food or water would cause him severe abdominal pain. Several imaging studies later, he underwent a cholecystectomy. This brought no lasting relief from his symptoms of nausea and vomiting, however. He was diagnosed with severe gastro-esophageal reflux which did not respond to any medications nor to feeds administered through a nasogastric tube. A transcutaneous J-tube was placed into his small intestine through the skin and all other feeding attempts stopped. J.B. was spitting out his own saliva, unable to tolerate swallowing, and began to believe that his tube feedings were causing severe headaches. He stopped even the tube feeds. By then he was taking only water through his tube and weighed 121 lbs (45% of his former weight).

When we saw J.B. at the Kartini Clinic he required transfer to the ICU because of life-threatening hypokalemia and hyponatremia: it was clear to us that he would likely have died in the night had his father not brought him in when he did. He had severe cognitive impairment and slow speech. Despite his age (18) we insisted that his father remain in Portland for family-based treatment

Once his fluid and electrolyte situation stabilized, olanzapine was initiated and then titrated to 7.5 mg/day. His anxiety began to abate. He had been paranoid and distrustful at first, but as he came to trust that we were there to help him, he relaxed more. Over time J.B. was able to take sips of water then of Boost ©. We discussed anxiety generated in the brain and its relationship to pain experienced in the stomach many times. By the third week he was able to eat solid food and the J-tube was removed. He was discharged to the DTU where his father and fiancée joined him to consolidate his progress in social eating. We were working on independent living skills and anxiety reduction with him when J.B.'s family removed him from treatment. He had gained about 20 lbs, his labs were normal, his speech clear, and his cognition appeared close to his reported baseline.

# 16.8　Discussion

The London experience, as described in *Eating Disorders: A Parents Guide*, is somewhat at variance to ours, in that we have given up treating this entity in an outpatient setting, believing that the much more prolonged course of outpatient treatment is often inefficient in restoring normal growth and development at a critical stage. Other providers, principally adult psychologists or psychiatrists, have reported their experience with outpatient treatment as well. Chorpita *et al.* [16] reported a 13-year-old girl whose "choking phobia" was treated with 14 sessions of behavioral and exposure techniques. Three case studies done in adults ages 33, 20 and 28 years, were reported by Ball, *et al.* [3]. They required 11-13 weekly sessions of between one and one and a half hours to treat successfully.

In our view 12 weeks is too long a time to wait for results in a young child who is wasted, whose growth is "on hold" and who may be dehydrated. It is furthermore not clear that the cognitive development of many younger patients will yield the same response to CBT and aversion techniques that it does in adults [78]. We prefer to treat aggressively either in the hospital or DTU those children who have lost enough weight to have fallen off their growth curve and are failing to thrive. The advantages of initial nasogastric feeds and fluids are the immediate control of fluid and electrolyte balance, the psychological relief of frightened and frustrated caretakers, and the emphasis on the non-volitional aspects of food phobia. This relieves guilt and reduces a child's conflict with their parents and extended family.

The multi-disciplinary team needed for family-based treatment to succeed is essential. At our institution, psychological and social consolidation takes place in the day treatment unit (DTU) where

the milieu therapists ensure that child and parents are both on
board with an eating plan that will establish good nutrition and
growth potential without any fears of choking or vomiting. Thus
we are able to promptly reverse weight and growth losses and
return the child to full functioning in a fraction of the time needed
for outpatient CBT/aversion/behavioral techniques. Once extinguished, our patients appear to resume normal life without further
eating problems. As with other childhood eating disorders, it is
hoped that early and aggressive treatment will improve outcome
and diminish morbidity.

## Clinical pearls

- Place a nasogastric tube to secure adequate intake.

- Families do a good job keeping their child alive until they
  can get help. Tell them so.

- Neuroleptic medication (olanzapine) is critical to success.

- Timing is everything—wait for medication, nutritional
  restoration, and the child's confidence in you as a provider
  before attempting to re-feed.

- Involve the parents, listen to them, and inspire their confidence.

# References

[1] American academy of pediatrics guidelines identifying and treating eating disorders. *Pediatrics*, 111(1):204–211, 2003.

[2] T. B. Baker et al. Current status and future prospects of clinical psychology toward a scientifically principled approach to mental and behavioral healthcare. *Psychological Science in the Public Interest*, 9(2), November 2002.

[3] S. G. Ball and M. W. Otto. Cognitive behavioral treatment of choking phobia: 3 case studies. *Psychother. Psychosom.*, 62:207–211, 1994.

[4] M. Barrera et al. The role of emotional social support in the psychological adjustment of siblings of children with cancer. *Child: Care, Health and Development*, 30(2):103–111, March 2004.

[5] L. Bellodi et al. Morbidity risk for obsessive-compulsive spectrum disorders in first-degree relatives of patients with eating disorders. *American Journal of Psychiatry*, 158(4):563–569, April 2001.

[6] D. H. Ben-Dor et al. Heritability, genetics and association findings in anorexia nervosa. *Israeli Journal of Psychiatry and Related Sciences*, 39(4):262–270, 2002.

[7] A. W. Bergen et al. Candidate genes for anorexia nervosa in the 1p33–36 linkage region: Serotonin 1D and delta opi-

oid receptor loci exhibit significant association to anorexia nervosa. *Molecular Psychiatry*, 8(4):397–406, April 2003.

[8]   S. Bordo. *Unbearable Weight*, page 171. Berkeley: University of California, 1993.

[9]   H. Bruch. Gaswechseluntersuchungen ueber die erholung nach arbeit bei einigen gesunden and kranken kindern [Gas exchange during rest after exertion in healthy and ill children]. *Jahrbuch fuer Kinderheilkunde*, 121:1–28, 1928.

[10]  H. Bruch. *Eating disorders*. Basic books, 4th edition, 1985.

[11]  C. M. Bulik, N. D. Berkman, K. A. Brownley, J. A. Sedway, and K.N. Lohr. Anorexia nervosa treatment: A systematic review of randomized controlled trials. *International Journal of Eating Disorders*, 40:310–320, 2007.

[12]  C. M. Bulik et al. The relation between eating disorders and components of perfectionism. *American Journal of Psychiatry*, 160(2):366–368, February 2003.

[13]  C. M. Bulik et al. Contemporary thinking about the role of genes and environment in eating disorders. *Epidemiologia e Psichiatria Sociale*, 13(2):91–98, April-June 2004.

[14]  C. M. Bulik and F. Tozzi. The genetics of bulimia nervosa. *Drugs Today (Barcelona, Spain)*, 40(9):741–749, September 2004.

[15]  E. Chen et al. Comparison of group and individual cognitive-behavioral therapy for patients with bulimia nervosa. *International Journal of Eating Disorders*, 33(3):241–254; discussion 255–256, April 2003.

[16] B. F. Chorpita, A. E. Vitali, and D. H. Barlow. Behavioral treatment of choking phobia in an adolescent: an experimental analysis. *Journal of Behavior Therapy and Experimental Psychiatry*, 28(4):307–315, 1997.

[17] C. Correll, P. Manu, V. Olshanskiy, et al. Cardiometabolic risk of second-generation antipsychotic medications during first time use in children and adolescents. *Journal of the American Medical Association*, 302(6):1765–1773, 2009.

[18] G. Deng and B. R. Cassileth. Integrative oncology: Complementary therapies for pain, anxiety, and mood disturbance. *CA: A Cancer Journal for Clinicians*, 55(2):109–116, March-April 2005.

[19] C. J. DeVile et al. Occult intracranial tumours masquerading as early onset anorexia nervosa. *British Medical Journal*, 311(7016):1359–1360, November 1995.

[20] M. Diaz-Marsa et al. A study of temperament and personality in anorexia and bulimia nervosa. *Journal of Personality Disorders*, 14(4):352–359, Winter 2000.

[21] I. Eisler et al. Family and individual therapy in anorexia nervosa: A 5-year follow-up. *Archives of General Psychiatry*, 54(11):1025–1030, November 1997.

[22] D. L. Elliot et al. Preventing substance use and disordered eating: Initial outcomes of the athena (athletes targeting healthy exercise and nutrition alternatives) program. *Archives of Pediatrics and Adolescent Medicine*, 158(11):1043–1049, November 2004.

[23]  E. Ernest.  Abdominal massage therapy for chronic constipation: A systematic review of controlled clinical trials. *Forschende Komplementarmedizin*, 6(3):149–151, June 1999.

[24]  S. Fassino et al.  Temperament and character in eating disorders: Ten years of studies. *Eating and Weight Disorders*, 9(2):81–90, June 2004.

[25]  A. Favaro et al. Total serum cholesterol and suicidality in anorexia nervosa. *Psychosomatic Medicine*, 66(4):548–552, July 2004.

[26]  M. M. Fichter and N. Quadflieg. Twelve-year course and outcome of bulimia nervosa. *Psychological Medicine*, 34(8):1395–1406, November 2004.

[27]  M. M. Fichter, N. Quadflieg, and S. Hedlund. Twelve-year course and outcome predictors of anorexia nervosa. *International Journal of Eating Disorders*, 39(2):87–100, march 1996.

[28]  M. Flament, C. Furino, and N. Godart. Psychopharmacology for eating disorders. *Evidence-Based Psychopharmacology*, pages 204–205, 2005.

[29]  G. K. Frank, U. F. Bailer, S. E. Henry, W. Drevets, C. Meltzer, J. Price, et al. Increased dopamine d2/d3 receptor binding after recovery from anorexia nervosa measured by positron emission tomography and raclopride. *Biological Psychiatry*, 58:908–912, 2005.

[30]  G. K. Frank et al. Neuroimaging studies in eating disorders. *CNS Spectrums*, 9(7):539–548, july 2004.

[31] S. Freud. On narcissism: Great books of the western world. *Chicago: Encyclopedia Britannica*, 54:401, 1982.

[32] D. Garner and P. Garfinkel. Hilde bruch. In *Handbook of Psychotherapy for Anorexia Nervosa and Bulimia*. New York: Guilford Press, 2nd edition, 1985.

[33] C. Gaser et al. Ventricular enlargement in schizophrenia related to volume reduction of the thalamus, striatum, and superior temporal cortex. *American Journal of Psychiatry*, 161(1):154–156, January 2004.

[34] J. Gelernter, G. Page, M. Stein, and S. Wood. Genome-wide linkage scan for loci predisposing to social phobia: Evidence for a chromosome 16 risk locus. *American Journal of Psychiatry*, 161(1):59–66, 2004.

[35] N. Godart et al. Are anxiety disorders more frequent in subjects with eating disorders? *Annales de Medecine Interne*, 154(4):209–218, September 2003.

[36] N. H. Golden. Osteopenia and osteoporosis in anorexia nervosa. *Adolescent Medicine*, 14(1):97–108, February 2003.

[37] N. H. Golden et al. Resumption of menses in anorexia nervosa. *Archives of Pediatrics and Adolescent Medicine*, 151(1):16–21, January 1997.

[38] N. H. Golden et al. Alendronate for the treatment of osteopenia in anorexia nervosa: a randomized, double-blind, placebo-controlled trial. *The Journal of Clinical Endocrinology and Metabolism*, 90(6):3179–3185, June 2005.

[39] N. H. Golden and W. Meyer. Nutritional rehabilitation of anorexia nervosa: Goals and dangers. *International Journal*

*of Adolescent Medicine and Health,* 16(2):131–144, April-June 2004.

[40] C. M. Gordon and L. M. Nelson. Amenorrhea and bone health in adolescents and young women. *Current Opinion in Obsterics and Gynecology,* 15(5):377–384, October 2003.

[41] P. Gorwood et al. The human genetics of anorexia nervosa. *European Journal of Pharmacology,* 480(1-3):163–70, November 2003.

[42] D. E. Grice et al. Evidence for a susceptibility gene for anorexia nervosa on chromosome 1. *American Journal of Human Genetics,* 70(3):787–792, March 2002.

[43] D. Grossmann et al. Cavernoma of the medulla oblongata mimicking 'anorexia nervosa'—a case report. *Klinische Paediatrie,* 214(1):41–44, January-February 2002.

[44] P. Hay et al. Individual psychotherapy in the outpatient treatment of adults with anorexia nervosa. *Cochrane Database of Systematic Reviews,* 4, 2003.

[45] R. B. Haynes, X. Yao, et al. Interventions to enhance medication adherence cochrane. *Cochrane Database of Systematic Reviews,* 4:CD000011, October 2005.

[46] D. B. Herzog et al. Mortality in eating disorders: A descriptive study. *International Journal of Eating Disorders,* 28(1):20–26, july 2000.

[47] H. W. Hoek. The incidence and prevalence of anorexia nervosa and bulimia nervosa in primary care. *Psychological Medicine,* 21(2):455–460, May 1991.

[48] B. A. Houtzager et al. Sibling self-report, parental proxies, and quality of life: The importance of multiple informants for siblings of a critically ill child. *Pediatric Hematology and Oncology*, 22(1):25–40, January-February 2005.

[49] K. Ikemoto et al. Number of striatal D-neurons is reduced in autopsy brains of schizophrenics. *Legal Medicine (Tokyo)*, 5(1):221–224, March 2003.

[50] S. Y. Jeon and H. Jung. The effects of abdominal meridian massage on constipation among cva patients. *Taehan Kanho Hakhoe Chi*, 35(1):135–142, February 2005.

[51] D. C. Jimerson and B. E. Wolfe. Neuropeptides in eating disorders. *CNS Spectrums*, 9(7):516–522, July 2004.

[52] J. Jordan et al. Anxiety and psychoactive substance use disorder comorbidity in anorexia nervosa or depression. *International Journal of Eating Disorders*, 34(2):211–209, September 2003.

[53] E. R. Kandel, J. H. Schwartz, and T. M. Jessell. Princibles of neural science: Third edition. *Appleton and Lange*, pages 5, 12, 1999.

[54] D. W. Kaplan et al. Identifying and treating eating disorders. *Pediatrics*, 111(1):204–211, January 2003.

[55] D. K. Katzman et al. Cognitive function and brain structure in females with a history of adolescent-onset anorexia nervosa. *Pediatrics*, 122(2):426–237, August 2008.

[56] W. H. Kaye et al. A search for susceptibility loci for anorexia nervosa: Methods and sample description. *Biological Psychiatry*, 47(9):794–803, May 2000.

[57] W. H. Kaye et al. Comorbidity of anxiety disorders with anorexia and bulimia nervosa. *American Journal of Psychiatry*, 161(12):2215–2221, December 2004.

[58] W. H. Kaye and B. Walsh. Psychopharmacology of eating disorders. *Neuropsychopharmacology: The Fifth Generation of Progress*, pages 1675–1683, 2002.

[59] A. Keys et al. *The Biology of Human Starvation*. University of Minnesota Press, 1950.

[60] R. M. Kliegman, R. E. Behrman, H. B. Jenson, and B. Stanton. *Nelson Textbook of Pediatrics*. Saunders, 17 edition, 2007.

[61] K. L. Klump et al. Temperament and character in women with anorexia nervosa. *The Journal of Nervous and Mental Disease*, 188(9):559–567, September 2000.

[62] K. L. Klump et al. The evolving genetic foundations of eating disorders. *The Psychiatric Clinics of North America*, 24(2):215–225, June 2001.

[63] K. L. Klump and K. Gobrogge. A review and primer of molecular genetic studies of anorexia nervosa. *International Journal of Eating Disorders*, 37:S43–S48, 2005.

[64] M. R. Kohn and N. H. Golden. Cardiac arrest and delirium: Presentations of the refeeding syndrome in severely malnourished adolescents with anorexia nervosa. *The Journal of Adolescent Health*, 22(3):239–243, March 1998.

[65] S. Kojima et al. Comparison of regional cerebral blood flow in patients with anorexia nervosa before and after weight gain. *Psychiatry Research*, 140(3):251–258, 2005.

[66] M. Koronyo-Hamaoui et al. CAG repeat polymorphism within the KCNN3 gene is a significant contributor to susceptibility to anorexia nervosa: A case-control study of female patients and several ethnic groups in the israeli jewish population. *American Journal of Medical Genetics Part B: Neuropsychiatric Genetics*, 131(1):76–80, November 2004.

[67] H. Kunugi et al. Low serum cholesterol in suicide attempters. *Biological Psychiatry*, 41(2):196–200, January 1997.

[68] B. Lask and R. Bryant. *Waugh Eeating Disorders: A Parent's Guide Revised Edition*. Brunner, 2004.

[69] D. Le Grange, R. Binford, and K. L. Loeb. Manualized family-based treatment for anorexia nervosa: A case series. *Journal of the American Academy of Child and Adolescent Psychiatry*, 44(1):41–46, January 2005.

[70] D. Le Grange, J. Lock, et al. Academy for eating disorders position paper: The role of the family in eating disorders. *International Journal of Eating Disorders*, 43(1):1–5, 2010.

[71] R. A. Lehman et al. Weight and height deficits in children with brain stem tumors. *Clinical Pediatrics*, 41(5):315–321, june 2002.

[72] B. E. Levin. Factors promoting and ameliorating the development of obesity. *Physiology and Behavior*, 86(5):633–669, December 2005.

[73] L. Lin et al. Brain tumor presenting as anorexia nervosa in a 19-year-old man. *Journal of the Formosan Medical Association*, 102(10):737–740, October 2003.

[74] Jim Locke. *Foreword to Eating with Your Anorexic, by Laura Collins.* New York: McGraw-Hills, 2005.

[75] J. D. Lundgren, S. Danoff-Burg, and D. A. Anderson. Cognitive-behavioral therapy for bulimia nervosa: an empirical analysis of clinical significance. *International Journal of Eating Disorders*, 35(3):262–274, April 2004.

[76] T. McFlarlane et al. Weight-related and shape-related self-evaluation in eating-disordered and non-eating-disordered women. *International Journal of Eating Disorders*, 29(3):328–335, April 2001.

[77] R. F. McKnight and R. J. Park. Atypical antipsychotics and anorexia nervosa: A review.

[78] R. McNally. Choking phobia: A review of the literature. *Comprehensive Psychiatry*, 39(1):83–89, 1994.

[79] P. Mehler. Diagnosis and care of patients with anorexia nervosa in primary care settings. *Annals of Internal Medicine*, 134(11):1048–1059, June 2001.

[80] C. Mika et al. Dietary treatment enhances bone formation in malnourished patients. *Journal of Gravitational Physiology*, 9(1):331–332, October 2002.

[81] D. Modan-Moses et al. Stunting of growth as a major feature of anorexia nervosa in male adolescents. In *Pediatrics*, volume 111, pages 270–276. February 2003.

[82] Richard Morton. *Phthisiologia or A Treatise of Consumption.* London, 2 edition, 1720.

[83] M. T. Munoz et al. The effects of estrogen administration on bone mineral density in adolescents with anorexia nervosa. *European Journal of Endocrinology*, 146(1):45–50, January 2002.

[84] K. M. Myers and M. S. Smith. Psychogenic polydipsia in a patient with anorexia nervosa. *Journal of Adolescent Health Care*, 6(5):404–406, September 1985.

[85] K. J. Neumarker. Mortality and sudden death in anorexia nervosa. *International Journal of Eating Disorders*, 21(3):205–212, January 1997.

[86] D. Nicholls, R. Chater, and B. Lask. Children into DSM don't go: A comparison of classification systems for eating disorders in childhood and early adolescence. *International Journal of Eating Disorders*, 28(3):317–324, November 2000.

[87] M. K. Nock. A multiple-baseline evaluation of the treatment of food phobia in a young boy. *Journal of Behavior Therapy and Experimental Psychiatry*, 33:217–225, 2002.

[88] R. M. Ornstein et al. Hypophosphatemia during nutritional rehabilitation in anorexia nervosa: Implications for refeeding and monitoring. *The Journal of Adolescent Health*, 32(1):83–88, January 2003.

[89] J. O'Toole. Personal communications with colleagues in Germany, Australia, and the United Kingdom.

[90] G. Patton et al. Abnormal eating attitudes in london school girls—a prospective epidemiological study. *Psychological Medicine*, 20(2):383–394, May 1990.

[91] K. J. Pederson, J. L. Roerig, and J. E. Mitchell. Towards the pharmacotherapy of eating disorders. *Expert Opinion on Pharmacotherapy*, 4(10):1659–1678, October 2003.

[92] T. Perreira et al. Role of therapeutic alliance in family therapy for adolescent anorexia nervosa. *International Journal of Eating Disorders*, 39(8):677–684, 2006.

[93] K. F. Phalen. Progress on lupus: New clarity for a baffling disease. *American Medical News*, 2002.

[94] R. Plomin et al. *Behavioral Genetics*, pages 246–247, 275. New York: Worth Publishers, 3 edition, 1997.

[95] G. Plumbo. Nutrition and healthy eating. `www.mayoclinic.com/health/caffeine/AN01211`, June, 2009.

[96] B. Ramot et al. The epidemiology of childhood acute lymphoblastic leukemia and non-Hodgkin's lymphoma in Israel between 1976 and 1981. In *Leukemia Research*, volume 8, pages 691–699. 1984.

[97] M. Ribases et al. Association of BDNF with restricting anorexia nervosa and minimum body mass index: a family-based association study of eight european populations. *European Journal of Human Genetics*, 13(4):428–434, April 2005.

[98] K. Richards et al. Use of complementary and alternative therapies to promote sleep in critically ill patients. *Critical Care Nursing Clinics of North America*, 15(3):329–340, September 2003.

[99] A. L. Robin et al. A controlled comparison of family versus individual therapy for adolescents with anorexia nervosa.

*Journal of the American Academy of Child and Adolescent Psychiatry*, 38(12):1482–1489, December 1999.

[100] J. Rutherford et al. Genetic influences on eating attitudes in a normal female twin population. *Psychological Medicine*, 23(2):425–236, May 1993.

[101] Menezes F. S. et al. Hypophosphatemia in critically ill children. *Revisto do Hospital das Clinicas do Faculdade de Medicina Sao Paulo*, 59(5):306–311, 2004.

[102] E. Salimei et al. Composition and characteristics of asses milk. *Animal Research*, 53(11):67–68, 2004.

[103] L. Serpell and J. Treasure. Bulimia nervosa: Friend or foe? the pros and cons of bulimia nervosa. *International Journal of Eating Disorders*, 32(2):164–170, September 2002.

[104] A. Shadaba et al. Re-feeding syndrome. *Journal of Laryngology and Otology*, 115(9):755–756, September 2001.

[105] I. Shai et al. Weight loss with a low-carbohydrate, mediterranean, or low-fat diet. *The New England Journal of Medicine*, 359(3):229–241, July 2008.

[106] T. Shamim et al. Resolution of vital sign instability: An objective measure of medical stability in anorexia nervosa. *Journal of Adolescent Health*, 32(1):73–77, January 2003.

[107] D. Sharpe and L. Rossiter. Siblings of children with a chronic illness: A meta-analysis. *Journal of Pediatric Psychology*, 27(8):699–710, December 2002.

[108] J. Siegel et al. Augmenting and reducing of visual evoked potentials in high- and low-sensation seeking humans, cats, and rats. *Behavior Genetics*, 27(6):557–563, November 1997.

[109] T. J. Silber. Eating disorders and health insurance. *Archives of Pediatrics and Adolescent Medicine*, 148(8):785–788, August 1994.

[110] L. A. Sim et al. Family-based therapy for adolescents with anorexia nervosa. *Mayo Clinic Proceedings*, 79(10):1305–1308, October 2004.

[111] L. T. Singer, B. Ambuel, S. Wade, and A. C. Jaffe. Cognitive-behavioral treatment of health- impairing food phobias in children. *Journal of the American Academy of Child and Adolescent Psychiatry*, 31:847–852, 1992.

[112] M. J. Sokol. Infection-triggered anorexia nervosa in children: Clinical description of four cases. *Journal of Child and Adolescent Psychopharmacology*, 10(2):133–145, Summer 2000.

[113] R. J. Sparks. *The papers of Hilde Bruch: A manuscript collection in the Harris County Medical Archive*. Number 7. Houston Academy of Medicine-Texas Medical Center Library, 1133 John Freeman Blvd. Houston, Texas 77030, 1985.

[114] M. Speranza et al. Current and lifetime prevalence of obsessive compulsive disorders in eating disorders. *L'Encephale*, 27(6):541–550, November-December 2001.

[115] S. Stahl. *Essential psychopharmacology*. Cambridge University Press, 3rd edition, 2008.

[116] E. A. Stamatakis and M. M. Hetherington. Neuroimaging in eating disorders. *Nutritional Neuroscience*, 6(6):325–334, December 2003.

[117] P. F. Sullivan, C. M. Bulik, and K. S. Kendler. Genetic epidemiology of binging and vomiting. *The British Journal of Psychiatry*, 173:75–79, November 1998.

[118] I. Swenne and P. T. Larsson. Heart risk associated with weight loss in anorexia nervosa and eating disorders: Risk factors for qtc interval prolongation and dispersion. *Acta Paediatrica*, 88(3):304–309, March 1999.

[119] T. Tadai et al. Body image changes in adolescents in development of self-rating body image (srbi) test and effects of sex, age and body shape. *The Japanese Journal of Psychiatry and Neurology*, 48(3):533–539, September 1994.

[120] G. Taubes. The soft science of dietary fat. *Science*, 291(5513):2536–2545, March 2001.

[121] J. L. Treasure and J. B. Owen. Intriguing links between animal behavior and anorexia nervosa. *International Journal of Eating Disorders*, 21(4):307–311, May 1997.

[122] M. Vervaet et al. Personality-related characteristics in restricting versus binging and purging eating disordered patients. *Comprehensive Psychiatry*, 45(1):37–43, September 2004.

[123] A. Wagner, H. Aizenstein, V. K. Venkatraman, J. Fudge, J. C. May, and L. andn others Mazurkewicz. Altered reward processing in women recovered from anorexia nervosa. *American Journal of Psychiatry*, 164:1842–1849, 2007.

[124] B. J. Walsch. Hypnotic alteration of body image in the eating disordered. *American Journal of Clinical Hypnosis*, 50(4):301–310, April 2008.

[125] G. T. Wilson et al. Cognitive-behavioral therapy for bulimia nervosa: Time course and mechanisms of change. *Journal of Consulting and Clinical Psychology*, 70(2):267–274, April 2002.

[126] M. D. Witting and K. Gallagher. Unique cutpoints for sitting-to-standing orthostatic vital signs. *American Journal of Emergency Medicine*, 21(1):45–47, January 2003.

[127] B. A. Woodruff. International emergency and refugee health branch, u.s. center for disease control and prevention arabella duffield. *ACC/SCN Secretariat*.

[128] B. D. Woodside and R. Staab. Management of psychiatric comorbidity in anorexia nervosa and bulimia nervosa. *CNS Drugs*, 20(8):655–663, 2006.

[129] Monika Woolsey. *Eating Disorders: A Clinical Guide to Counseling and Treatment American Dietetic Association*. Chicago, 2002.

[130] J. Yager et al. Practice guideline for the treatment of patients with eating disorders (revision). american psychiatric association work group on eating disorders. *American Journal of Psychiatry*, 157(1):1–39, January 2000.

# Appendix A

## R.E.D.S.-C.

**RATING OF EATING DISORDER SEVERITY (R.E.D.S.):** **The scores on this interview may be a combination of answers obtained directly from the child and report by the parent.**

Interviewer: _____ Date: _____

Present at interview: _____

Patient Name: _____ Age: ___ years ___ months   D.O.B. _____

□ Female   □ Male        Tanner stage: B: _____   PH: _____

School name: _____   Grade _____

| R.E.D.S. – Child Score: |
| Confidence Score: |

## 1.    INADEQUATE FOOD INTAKE

Tell me a little about yourself; give me "a day in the life"…when do you get up?  What is your routine?  Are you ever do busy that you skip breakfast?  What do you eat exactly…not in the last week…but in the few weeks before last week? Which classes are you taking? (younger children: do you have recess?)  Who do you eat lunch with?  Do you bring it or buy it?  What do you eat?  Who is home when you get home from school?  Do you have a snack? Are you hungry? How much homework do you have? Do you hang out with your friends after school? Who cooks dinner?  What do YOU typically prefer to have? (If patient binges, estimate calories on binge day/non-binge day and obtain an average of calories/day)

0. Eats adequate amounts to reach or maintain normal body weight.
1. Occasionally eats less than adequate amounts.
2. Often eats less than adequate amounts.
3. Consistently eats inadequate amounts (but at least 1000 kcal/day).
4. Consistent marked inadequacy of caloric intake (but at least 500 kcal/day).
5. Severe caloric restriction (average intake less than 500 kcal/day).

| CONFIDENCE RATING: (Mark one) | Little/No Confidence | Significant Doubts | Mild Doubts | Moderate Confidence | Strong Confidence |
|---|---|---|---|---|---|
| | ❏ 0 | ❏ 1 | ❏ 2 | ❏ 3 | ❏ 4 |

## 2.   DIMINISHED FOOD RANGE

Tell me about what you like to eat.  Do you eat red meat? (for younger children: do you like hamburgers? Pork chops?) Can you eat chicken or turkey? Fish? Do you drink milk? Does it have to be fat free or skim? How about cheese? Yogurt? Does it have to be fat free?  Do you like pasta like spaghetti? Bread? Rice? Muffins? Do you eat cookies? Did you used to before your eating changed? Cake? Ice cream? Do you ever dream about food? What food appears in your dreams?   Summary:

- ❑       red meat (e.g., pork, lamb, beef)
- ❑       poultry
- ❑       catch fish/shellfish
- ❑       milk/cheese/yogurt
- ❑       fruit/vegetables
- ❑       grains (e.g., bread, muffins, cereal, rice, pasta)
- ❑       desserts (e.g., pie, cake, ice cream)

(NOTE:  When rating this item, do not include food that is purged) **THE FOLLOWING ARE SOME GUIDELINES IN DETERMINING DEGREE OF RESRICTING:**

0.  No restriction of food types whatever.
1.  No restriction apart from fat content
2.  Mild limitation (perhaps has eaten from at least 5 of the above-listed food categories).
3.  Moderate limitation (perhaps has eaten from at least 4 of the above-listed food categories).
4.  Marked limitation (perhaps has only eaten from 3 of the above-listed food categories).
5.  Severe restriction of food types (has eaten fewer than 3 of the above-listed food categories).

| CONFIDENCE RATING: (Mark one) | Little/No Confidence | Significant Doubts | Mild Doubts | Moderate Confidence | Strong Confidence |
|---|---|---|---|---|---|
| | ❑ 0 | ❑ 1 | ❑ 2 | ❑ 3 | ❑ 4 |

## 3.   DISCOMFORT WHEN EATING IN PUBLIC

Tell me where you like to eat. Are you comfortable eating with your friends? (Ask specifically about members of the opposite sex). Do you prefer to eat at home?  In your room?  Is there anyone you don't like to eat with? Do you ever avoid going somewhere because you know people will be eating there? Do you like parties where food is served?

0.  Complete comfort when eating in public
1.  Small degree of uneasiness when eating in public or around certain people
2.  Sometimes avoids eating in public due to discomfort
3.  Often avoids eating in public due to discomfort
4.  Mostly avoids eating in public due to discomfort
5.  Always eats alone due to discomfort.

| CONFIDENCE RATING: (Mark one) | Little/No Confidence | Significant Doubts | Mild Doubts | Moderate Confidence | Strong Confidence |
|---|---|---|---|---|---|
| | ❑ 0 | ❑ 1 | ❑ 2 | ❑ 3 | ❑ 4 |

## 4.  BINGE QUANTITY

Do you know what a binge is?
There are two kinds of binges that sometimes happen to people.
One is where you get really, really hungry or bored and you go in the kitchen or take food out of the kitchen and eat a whole lot---more than you normally ever eat, like the whole bag of chips or the carton of ice cream.(Objective binge)  Then you feel bad.  Does that ever happen to you?
The other kind of binge is what we call the "rule breaking binge" where you don't eat a lot of food-it might even be just a grape, but you feel bad because it has broken a rule or a goal you set for yourself, like "I won't eat before nighttime" or "I will only eat carrots and celery today".
Has that ever happened to you? (Subjective binge)

0.  Has not had subjective or objective binge episodes this month.
1.  Subjective binge episodes only (binge eating is confined to small amounts).
2.  Binges consist of amounts of food just large enough to be considered objective binge episodes.
3.  Objective binges consisting of large amounts of food.
4.  Objective binges consisting of extremely large amounts of food.
5.  Objective binges consisting of such enormous amounts of food that stomach rupture is at risk.

| CONFIDENCE RATING: (Mark one) | Little/No Confidence | Significant Doubts | Mild Doubts | Moderate Confidence | Strong Confidence |
|---|---|---|---|---|---|
| | ❏ 0 | ❏ 1 | ❏ 2 | ❏ 3 | ❏ 4 |


## 5.  OBJECTIVE BINGE FREQUENCY

(Having established which of the two binge types the patient suffers from, you now ask....)
In the last 3 months, how often has this happened to you?

0.  No objective binge episodes.
1.  Binge episodes less than twice per week (on average).
2.  Binge episodes twice a week or more, but less than daily (on average).
3.  Binge episodes at least daily, but less than twice per day (on average).
4.  Binge episodes at least twice daily, but less than four times per day (on average).
5.  Binge episodes four or more times per day (on average).

| CONFIDENCE RATING: (Mark one) | Little/No Confidence | Significant Doubts | Mild Doubts | Moderate Confidence | Strong Confidence |
|---|---|---|---|---|---|
| | ❏ 0 | ❏ 1 | ❏ 2 | ❏ 3 | ❏ 4 |

## 6.  PURGE METHOD

Have you ever felt so bad about what you have eaten that you felt sick to your stomach and threw it all up?  Do you ever throw up to make yourself feel better?  Have you ever taken any medicines to help you throw up? Have you ever stuck anything down your throat to make yourself throw up?  Have you ever taken pills or medicines to help you get rid of calories or lose weight?  Have you ever taken anything to help you go to the bathroom more often?
(NOTE:  We define purging as the use of any of the above methods with the intent of eliminating food or preventing absorption of calories ("purging with exercise" covered elsewhere).

0.  Has never used any method to purge
1.  Purged only by vomiting once or twice or tried laxatives once or twice, but "didn't like it and stopped".
2.  Purges consistently or frequently only by vomiting or **one** other method (e.g. laxatives)
3.  Purges consistently or frequently by two methods (e.g. vomiting and laxatives)
4.  Purges consistently or frequently by two methods whereby one of the methods involves using syrup of ipecac or insulin manipulation

| CONFIDENCE RATING: (Mark one) | Little/No Confidence | Significant Doubts | Mild Doubts | Moderate Confidence | Strong Confidence |
|---|---|---|---|---|---|
| | ❏ 0 | ❏ 1 | ❏ 2 | ❏ 3 | ❏ 4 |

## 7.  PURGE FREQUENCY

In the last 3 months, how often do you find yourself throwing up or taking medicine to try and take away some of the food you have eaten? (average over the last 3 months)

0.  Never
1.  Purged, but less than twice per week (on average).
2.  Purged twice per week or more, but less than daily (on average).
3.  Purged at least daily, but less than twice per day (on average).
4.  Purged at least daily, but less than four times per day (on average).
5.  Purged four times per day or more (on average).

| CONFIDENCE RATING: (Mark one) | Little/No Confidence | Significant Doubts | Mild Doubts | Moderate Confidence | Strong Confidence |
|---|---|---|---|---|---|
| | ❏ 0 | ❏ 1 | ❏ 2 | ❏ 3 | ❏ 4 |

## 8. FREQUENCY OF COMPULSIVE OR COMPENSATORY EXERCISE

Some people feel bad if they can't exercise everyday…or if they feel they have eaten too much. Does that ever happen to you?

I understand that you may be interested in being active and fit…is that true? What kinds of things do you do to try and stay fit and get healthy? How about for fun? Do you ever get up early in the morning to work out? How about late at night, especially when you can't sleep? Do you ever do exercise videos? jumping jacks? Crunches? How many can you do? Do you ever try to make up for eating by "exercising it off"?

On average over the last 3 months, the patient has:

0. Not exercised compensatorily or compulsively
1. Compensatory or compulsive exercise episodes, but less than twice per week (on average).
2. Compensatory or compulsive exercise episodes, twice per week or more, but less than daily (on average).
3. Compensatory or compulsive exercise episodes daily, but less than twice per day (on average).
4. Compensatory or compulsive exercise episodes twice a day or more, but less than four times per day (on average).
5. Compensatory or compulsive exercise episodes four times per day or more (on average).

| CONFIDENCE RATING: (Mark one) | Little/No Confidence | Significant Doubts | Mild Doubts | Moderate Confidence | Strong Confidence |
|---|---|---|---|---|---|
| | ❏ 0 | ❏ 1 | ❏ 2 | ❏ 3 | ❏ 4 |

## 9.    ABNORMALLY LOW BODY MASS INDEX

HEIGHT: _____          WEIGHT: _____

(NOTE:  Body Mass Index (BMI) can be calculated by multiplying the weight in pounds by 700 and dividing by the height in inches squared.

$$BMI = \frac{weight\ (Lbs)\ x\ 703}{ht.\ (inches)\ x\ ht.\ (inches)}$$

0 = BMI at or above 50 % tile for age
1 = BMI between 25% tile and 49 %tile for age
2 = BMI between 10% tile and 24%tile for age
3 = BMI between 3% and 9% tile
4 = BMI below < 3% tile

CONFIDENCE RATING:
Automatically mark "4" strong confidence

Body Mass Index Graph

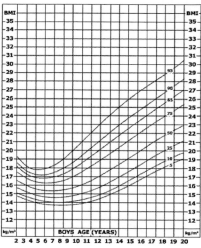
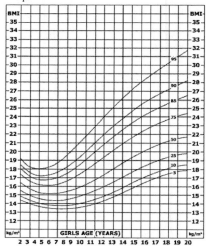

## 10. SEVERITY OF WEIGHT LOSS

IBW:
(girls) = 100 # for 5 ft. and 5 # for each subsequent inch in height
(boys) = 106# for 5 ft. and 6 # for each subsequent inch in height

**IF PATIENT BEGAN ILLNESS ABOVE CALCULATED IDEAL BODY WEIGHT USE % PREMORBID WEIGHT NOT % IBW**

Do you have any idea what you weigh today? (Don't reveal weight) How do you feel about this weight? If I had a magic wand and could make you any weight in the whole world, what weight would be too low for you—I mean, pick a weight that is so low you would be scared to weight so little. (Then mention a number a few pounds below the one they pick) what if you weighed ___, would that be ok? (If no) What would you do if you weighed that much? So what weight would be too much for you? And what would be just right? * if unable to answer code "0" and mark with "little or no confidence"

0.  Can accept a weight 91% of IBW or greater **OR** pre-morbid weight.
1.  Wants to be at a weight 85-90%of IBW **OR** pre-morbid weight.
2.  Wants to be at a weight 80-85% of IBW **OR** pre-morbid weight.
3.  Wants to be at a weight 75-80% of IBW **OR** pre-morbid weight.
4.  Wants to be at a weight 70-75% of IBW **OR** pre-morbid weight.
5.  Wants to be at a weight less than 70% IBW **OR** pre-morbid weight.

| CONFIDENCE RATING: (Mark one) | Little/No Confidence | Significant Doubts | Mild Doubts | Moderate Confidence | Strong Confidence |
|---|---|---|---|---|---|
| | ❏ 0 | ❏ 1 | ❏ 2 | ❏ 3 | ❏ 4 |


## 11. COGNITIVE DRIVE FOR THINNESS

Since your parents have brought you here because of concerns about weight, I wonder whether you are concerned about your weight yourself?

0.  Able to see herself/himself as needing to gain weight or maintain weight within healthy parameters.
1.  Not sure about needing to gain weight, wants guidance.
2.  Does not want to gain weight to 90-100% IBW or pre-morbid wt. (which may have been "high")
3.  Strongly antagonistic to gaining weight even to 85% IBW or premorbid wt.
4.  Does not want to *gain* weight at all despite the need for restricting to maintain current wt.
5.  Not only refuses to gain weight at all, but insists she/he needs to *lose* weight regardless of any health consequences to weight loss.

| CONFIDENCE RATING: (Mark one) | Little/No Confidence | Significant Doubts | Mild Doubts | Moderate Confidence | Strong Confidence |
|---|---|---|---|---|---|
| | ❏ 0 | ❏ 1 | ❏ 2 | ❏ 3 | ❏ 4 |

## 12. PREOCCUPATION WITH SHAPE OR WEIGHT

I imagine there has been a lot of talk going on at your house about weight, shape and food, right? Some kids tell me that at first they didn't think about food and weight a lot, but that gradually they came to think about it all the time—sometimes so much so that it's even hard to concentrate at school. Has that happened to you?

    0. Infrequent or absent thoughts about shape or weight.
    1. Frequent thoughts about shape or weight (but not present daily).
    2. Frequent thoughts about shape or weight (at least daily).
    3. Preoccupation with thoughts about shape or weight, can't help talking about it sometimes and comparing other kids to themselves.
    4. Obsession with thoughts about shape or weight, compares everyone to him/herself all of the time.
    5. Obsessed with thoughts about shape or weight to the exclusion of almost all other thoughts (difficulty with concentration).

| CONFIDENCE RATING: (Mark one) | Little/No Confidence | Significant Doubts | Mild Doubts | Moderate Confidence | Strong Confidence |
|---|---|---|---|---|---|
| | ❏ 0 | ❏ 1 | ❏ 2 | ❏ 3 | ❏ 4 |

## 13. BODY IMAGE DISTURBANCE

How are you feeling today about your own body? Do you feel you are too thin? Just right? Somewhat too big in places? Too fat?
(If answers the later two) Let's be specific: how satisfied are you with the shape of your stomach, hips, thighs? How comfortable have you been when you look at yourself in a full length mirror? How comfortable are you in a bathing suit? When was the last time you wore one?

    0. No *inappropriate* dissatisfaction, e.g. "I guess I'm ok" or "I'm too skinny" (when this is an appropriate observation) **OR** "I'm still too big" (when they are still technically overweight).
    1. Mild body image dissatisfaction, e.g. "I'm not really happy with my size/shape: or "I could be thinner somewhere, I guess."
    2. Moderate body image dissatisfaction *or* distortion, e.g. "I'm too fat in the stomach" when this is clearly not true.
    3. Global body dissatisfaction ("I hate my body") **or** distortion ("I'm too fat" when clearly not true)
    4. Global body dissatisfaction ("I hate my body") **and** distortion ("I'm too fat" when clearly not true)
    5. Delusionally obsessed with large size of body in spite of emaciation and/or engaged in the delusional belief that others are perceiving them as fatter than everyone else

| CONFIDENCE RATING: (Mark one) | Little/No Confidence | Significant Doubts | Mild Doubts | Moderate Confidence | Strong Confidence |
|---|---|---|---|---|---|
| | ❏ 0 | ❏ 1 | ❏ 2 | ❏ 3 | ❏ 4 |

**14. DENIAL OF SERIOUSNESS OF WT. LOSS/ FAILURE TO GAIN WT.**

I understand that you have lost weight and that everyone is concerned about this, how do you feel about your weight loss? Did you want to come to the doctor's? How would you feel about the clinic helping you stop the weight loss and gain some back? Did you know that weight loss can affect the heart? Cause hair to fall out? Stop your growth in height? Stop your periods from coming (for girls)?

0. Has not lost more than a few pounds and has no plans to do so.
1. Generally believes their wt. loss/failure to gain appropriately is not a problem, but willing to listen to advice to the contrary
2. Firmly believes that there are no negative consequences to their own weight loss/ abnormally low body weight, or understands that there may be in the future, but are nonetheless unwilling to comply with weight gain.
3. Firmly believes there are no negative consequences to weight loss/abnormally low body weight despite moderate complications (e.g. amenorrhea, always cold) or understands that there may be, but are nonetheless unwilling to comply with weight gain.
4. Firmly believes there are no negative consequences to weight loss or abnormally low body weight despite severe complications (e.g. hospitalization, edema, heart problems, electrolyte disturbances)

| CONFIDENCE RATING: (Mark one) | Little/No Confidence | Significant Doubts | Mild Doubts | Moderate Confidence | Strong Confidence |
|---|---|---|---|---|---|
| | ❑ 0 | ❑ 1 | ❑ 2 | ❑ 3 | ❑ 4 |

**15. SOCIAL IMPACT**

(You may need the parent's input on this issue, especially with very young children.)
I'm wondering whether or not all this bother and talk about food has made you feel differently about doing things with your friends? Do you hang out with your friends ("play with your friends", in a younger child) as much as you used to? Are you spending more time alone doing your homework than you used to?

0. No social problem associated with eating disorder.
1. Mild impairment in social relationships, more alone time
2. Moderate social impairment, not calling friends or going places with them
3. Moderate social impairment, has been noticed by school teacher/others outside of family.
4. Marked social impairment, little interaction with former friends/schoolmates
5. Severe social impairment, unable to attend school or needing to be home schooled.

| CONFIDENCE RATING: (Mark one) | Little/No Confidence | Significant Doubts | Mild Doubts | Moderate Confidence | Strong Confidence |
|---|---|---|---|---|---|
| | ❑ 0 | ❑ 1 | ❑ 2 | ❑ 3 | ❑ 4 |

## 16.    PHYSICAL IMPACT

Now I have some medical questions for you.

Have you noticed that you feel colder than you used to, or that you are cold when other people feel normal or warm? Have you had to wear more clothes to stay warm, especially at night?
Have you had headaches? Stomachaches?
Have you felt dizzy or faint? Had "black-out" spells?
Have you had less energy to do sports or exercise?
Have you ever had a period? When was your last normal seeming period? Have you had any lighter-than-usual-seeming periods?
Have you had chest pain or shortness of breath? Heart racing?
When was the last time you changed shoe sizes?
Do you ever have trouble having bowel movements ("pooping" for a younger child)?
Do you have a hard time falling asleep at night? Do you wake up often during the night?
Do you ever wet the bed? (if yes) Is this new?
Are your hands or feet swollen or puffy during the day?
Have you noticed your skin is drier than it used to be? How about your scalp and hair?
Is your hair falling out?
Do you find yourself drinking a lot of fluids during the day? How about caffeinated beverages?
Have you noticed you bruise more easily than you used to?
Do cuts, scrapes and burns take longer to heal?

0.  No physical impairment associated with eating disorder.
1.  Mild physical symptoms associated with eating disorder (e.g., fatigue, lassitude, coldness).
2.  Moderate physical symptom (one only) associated with eating disorder (e.g., syncope (fainting), amenorrhea, bowel problems).
3.  Moderate physical symptoms (two or more) associated with eating disorder (e.g., syncope and amenorrhea, constipation and insomnia, etc.).
4.  Major illnesses or complications requiring medical intervention (e.g., dehydration, electrolyte abnormalities, chest pain, black-out spells, edema, new onset enuresis) OR PATIENT CURENTLY MEETS HOSPITALIZATION CRITERIA
5.  Major illness or complication which is life-threatening (e.g., renal failure, cardiac failure) OR PATIENT HAS BEEN ADMITTED TO THE ICU

| CONFIDENCE RATING: (Mark one) | Little/No Confidence | Significant Doubts | Mild Doubts | Moderate Confidence | Strong Confidence |
|---|---|---|---|---|---|
| | ❏ 0 | ❏ 1 | ❏ 2 | ❏ 3 | ❏ 4 |

| DIRECTIONS FOR OBTAINING TOTAL SCORE | DIRECTIONS FOR OBTAINING CONFIDENCE SCORE |
|---|---|

DIRECTIONS FOR OBTAINING TOTAL SCORE

Add scores of Scales 1 through 16 for total score

DIRECTIONS FOR OBTAINING CONFIDENCE SCORE

Confidence ratings are coded from 0 (little or no confidence) to 4 (strong confidence). Confidence score is calculated by adding all confidence ratings.

1. Inadequate Food Intake        ____   ____
2. Diminished Food Range         ____   ____
3. Discomfort When Eating in Public   ____   ____
4. Binge Quantity                ____   ____
5. Objective Binge Frequency     ____   ____
6. Purge Method                  ____   ____
7. Purge Frequency               ____   ____
8. Frequency Of Compulsive Exercise   ____   ____
9. Abnormally Low Body Mass Index    ____   ____
10. Severity of Weight Loss      ____   ____
11. Cognitive Drive For Thinness    ____   ____
12. Preoccupation With Shape Or Weight   ____   ____
13. Body Image Disturbance       ____   ____
14. Denial of Seriousness/Failure to Gain   ____   ____
15. Social Impact                ____   ____
16. Physical Impact              ____   ____

| **Total Score of possible 80** | | | **Confidence Score of possible 64** | |
|---|---|---|---|---|

## INSTRUCTIONS FOR INTERVIEWERS

The REDS-child is a rating scale adapted from Dr. Goldner's original R.E.D.S. for use with children and teens under age 17 with eating disorders (anorexia nervosa, bulimia nervosa, and related disorders).

All sixteen ratings are to be completed during an interview with the patient/subject  However, the interviewer should use additional questions and any other available information (e.g. observed eating behaviors, parental information) in order to derive the most accurate rating possible for each of the sixteen items. In each item, **choose only one number** (from 0 to 5) which appears most accurate. In a situation where it cannot be determined which of two numbers is most accurate, choose the lower number.

In addition, a confidence rating is required for each of the sixteen items. The confidence rating indicates the level of confidence that the interview estimates in the rating for each item. Choose only one confidence rating in each item and choose the lesser level of confidence in a situation where it cannot be determined which of two confidence ratings is most accurate.

**In order to achieve maximum accuracy in rating item #9 (Abnormal Body Mass Index), a weight scale and height measure should be used in a patient with only a gown, but no other clothing.**
Permission to reproduce or employ the R.E.D.S. for clinical or research purposes must be obtained by contacting:

Dr. Elliot M. Goldner
Eating Disorders Clinic
St. Paul's Hospital
1081 Burrard Street
Vancouver, B.C. Canada V6Z 1Y6

# Appendix B

*Kartini Clinic, P.C.*

2800 N. Vancouver, Suite 118
Portland, Oregon 97227
Phone (503) 249-8851   Fax (503) 282-3409
www.kartiniclinic.com

## FAMILY HISTORY QUESTIONNAIRE FOR PARENTS

Patient's Name: _____   Date of appointment: ___/___/____
Current age: _____   Primary care physician: _____
Date of Birth: _____

### HISTORY OF PRESENT ILLNESS

Who is filling out this form?

Please list all providers your child has seen for eating problems:

When and what was done?

How did you feel about that treatment?

**Who referred you to Kartini Clinic?**

When and how did your child's problems with food begin?

Was the onset of your child's symptoms sudden (within a few days) following an acute infection of any kind?

What about your child's eating problems have you most frightened or concerned?

Briefly describe your family's eating style and <u>who prepares</u>:

Breakfast?

Lunch?

Dinner?

Who is home after school when your child gets home?

How many times a week do you eat dinner at the table together?

How many times do you eat out per week?

Who does the grocery shopping?

Does your family keep Kosher?

Does your family eat vegetarian food only?

Are there other food restrictions your family follows?

What are your family's schedules like everyday including work hours?

To your knowledge, has your child ever taken diet pills? Laxatives? Ipecac? Water pills?

How do you find your child's weight at this point? How was it before the eating disorder started?

To your knowledge does your child ever get rid of any food by vomiting?

Does he/she ever binge (eat very large quantities of food at a time)?

To your knowledge, what is the most your child has weighed?

To your knowledge, what is the least your child has weighed at current height?

## PREVIOUS MEDICAL HISTORY

Where was your child born?  City_____    State_____    Country_____

Birth weight? _____ Premature?_____ Over-due?_____ On time?_____
Do you remember your Apgar Score?      What was it? _____  _____

Where did you live for the year before you got pregnant?

How old were you at the time of birth?

How many pregnancies had you had before?        Live births?

Did you have any complications?

<u>During Pregnancy</u> (please circle any that apply or write in your own)

Bleeding      High blood pressure      Diabetes     Anemia        Toxemia

Pre-eclampsia    Seizures     Blood clots       Placenta problems        Early water break

Fever     Depression     Psychological Stress      Exposure to toxins/infections/substances

Other (please be specific)_____

<u>During Birth</u> (please circle any that apply or write in your own)

Cesarian section (C-Section)       Cord around neck     Very large baby     Small baby

Bleeding       Oxygen needed        Forceps needed        Breech birth          Fetal Distress

Other (please be specific)_____

<u>Postpartum – after delivery</u> (please circle any that apply or write in your own)

Low temperature      Jaundice      Tremors      Seizures       Limpness

Poor feeding   NICU (Intensive care/Special nursery)       Depression in mother

Other (please be specific)_____

Had you been on a diet of any kind before you got pregnant?    During your pregnancy?

Did you take any medication before your pregnancy?       During your pregnancy?

Was your child breast fed?        For how long was she/he breast fed?

How easy was he/she to feed as a small child?

Any history of strep throat?

Has he/she had any major illnesses, surgeries or hospitalizations?

**Is she/he allergic to any medications?** _____

**Is she/he allergic to any foods?** _____
List any medications your child is currently taking, including vitamins, homeopathic or herbal preparations:

Do you recall anything unusual about your child's motor development (walking, crawling, coordination)?

Fine motor development (handling a spoon and other small tools such as a crayon or pencil)?

Language development?

Social development?

To your knowledge, does your child smoke cigarettes? Drink alcohol? Take drugs?

**If a girl,** when did she start her periods?          When was her last period?

About how much did she weigh at the time of her last period?

When did her mother start her periods?

Her sisters?

**If a boy,** when did he start to go through puberty?
Was he earlier/later/the same as his friends?

When did his dad start puberty?          Was he earlier/later/the same as his friends?

To your knowledge, has your child ever had sex, voluntarily or involuntarily? If involuntarily, when did this occur and has this been reported to child protective services and/or to the police?

Has your child ever had psychological testing done? When? By whom?

Has your child ever seen a psychiatrist or therapist?
If yes, what was the reason your child saw a psychiatrist and/or therapist?

Were you included in the therapy sessions or kept informed of progress?

When was the last time your child saw the therapist?

Has your child ever taken a medication for attention, concentration, depression, insomnia or stress? (please list):

Who prescribed the medication?

Do you give this medication or does your child take it themselves?

Has your child ever displayed any self-injurious behavior like cutting or high-risk behavior that lead to some kind of injury?

Has your child ever discussed suicide, made a suicide attempt, and/or been hospitalized for suicidal thoughts and/or suicidal behavior? If your child has been hospitalized: When? For how long? More than once?

## FAMILY HISTORY

**Family medical history is very important; if you have time you might want to ask your relatives some of these questions since not everyone knows everyone else's medical history.**

The following are the people whose history we would like to know. The conditions we would like to know about are listed on *page 7*. The easiest way to fill out this part is to *lay the list of possible conditions next to the list of family members* and as you read through the list of conditions write in any that pertain next to the family member's name. *Please give height and approximate weight).*

- **Patient's mother – Height: _____Weight: _____**

- **Patient's father – Height: _____Weight: _____**

- **Patient's sisters (height and weight)**

- **Patient's brothers (height and weight)**

- **Patient's first cousins (height and weight)**

- **Maternal grandmother (patient's mother's mother) – Height: _____Weight: _____**

- **Maternal grandfather (patient's mother's father) – Height: _____Weight: _____**

- **Maternal uncles and aunts (patient's mother's brothers and sisters) (ht and wt)**

- **Paternal grandmother (patient's father's mother) – Height: _____Weight: _____**

- **Paternal grandfather (patient's father's father) – Height: _____Weight: _____**

- **Paternal uncles and aunts (patient's father's brothers and sisters)**

**List of possible conditions (<u>and any other you might think of</u>) for you to write in next to the person's name on pages 5 and 6:**

- A history of heart attacks or other heart problems
- A family member who died suddenly under age 50
- Joint problems
- Someone with attention deficit disorders or related problems
- A history of weight problems
- A history of many diets
- A history of food allergies
- Currently on a diet
- Food fads
- A person who eats only a very narrow range of foods
- A person who cannot stand to have their food touching on the plate
- A person who is a fanatic exerciser
- A person who seems overly concerned with their appearance
- A person who seems overly concerned about other people's body size and shape
- A history of anorexia
- A period of time when they lost a lot of weight
- A history of bulimia
- A history of panic attacks
- Someone who washes their hands many, many times
- Someone who is afraid of germs
- A history of sleep disorders such as insomnia, nightmares, night terrors or sleep walking
- A history of anxiety, who might be afraid of unusual things such as meeting people or going outside
- A person who must have everything <u>very</u> tidy
- Who must have their closet color coded
- A person for whom certain numbers have special or magical significance
- A person who cannot leave the house without checking on things may times
- A person in the family who has been in a hospital for a mental illness
- Someone with learning disabilities or difficulties
- Someone with tics
- A person with diabetes
- A person with high blood pressure
- Children who died in infancy or childhood
- Someone that may have a problem with alcohol or drugs
- Depression, Seasonal affective disorder or Bipolar disorder (manic depression)
- Schizophrenia
- Autoimmune diseases such as lupus
- Rheumatoid arthritis, Rheumatic fever, M.S. or Thyroid illness
- High cholesterol
- Cancer. If so, what kind?
- Anyone who has taken medications to help them with mental or emotional problems or to control stress
- A person who has committed or attempted suicide
- Someone who 'binges' or eats huge amounts of food in one sitting
- Someone who vomits to control their weight
- A 'worrier'
- Premenstrual Syndrome (PMS)
- Someone who fits the description "perfectionistic"

**SOCIAL HISTORY**
Who lives at home now?  If siblings are not living at home, where are they living?


Please list all full biological siblings with gender and date of birth


Please list all half biological siblings with gender and date of birth (identify if on mother's or father's side)


Age of parents?

Parent's occupation, employer, and job contentment?


Dominant Family Values? i.e. educational achievement, financial success, humanitarian, religion.


How long have you (parents) been together?  _____  If not married, what is the nature of your relationship?  If divorced, how long?


Parents' previous marriages:


How would you describe your marital/parental relationship?  If divorced or separated, describe your custody arrangement and parenting plan:


How do parents communicate with each other?  What did each of you learn about parenting and communication from your respective families of origin?


Parenting styles, including similarities and differences:

How do family members communicate with each other?

How are decisions made in your family?

How are conflicts handled in your family?

Has anyone in the family spent time in jail or prison? Or ever been in trouble with the Law?

Does your family have a religious affiliation you would like us to know about?

Is your child involved in a religious or other social group?

List any diets family members may currently be on:

Are there any particular family issues bothering parents or your child presently?

Recent family stressors or challenges?

Parenting styles, similarities and differences?

Sibling rivalry or other issues?

What are your family strengths?

## ACADEMIC HISTORY

What grade level? _____     Which school does your child attend?

What is their academic record like?

Does your child have a job outside of school?

Has your child ever had difficulties learning school material?

What has been their best subject or most favored interest or hobby?

Is your child involved in sports, music or art?

Would you describe your child as (circle all that apply)?

Outgoing and social   Introverted, but social        Shy, but has friends        A loner

Has there been a difference in your child's social life since the eating disorder began?

What are the three best character traits of your child?

1) _____

2) _____

3) _____

# Appendix C

## Legacy Emanuel Children's Hospital
Eating Disorder Hospital Protocol
Privilege System Phase I
**Critical Medical Bedrest in ICU**

**Activity:**
- ✓ Patients at this phase are on critical medical bedrest and are to remain in bed at all times.
- ✓ **No Excursions** allowed at this phase.

**Room:**
- ✓ Room temperature to be set at 75-80°F at all times.

**Bathroom/Hygiene:**
- ✓ Bathroom privileges are by bedpan only.
- ✓ May sponge bath in bed.
- ✓ May brush teeth in bed.
- ✓ Sweatshirt and long pants to be worn when outside of room.

**Meals:**
- ✓ Food is regarded as medicine for our purposes, and nursing staff and the patients will follow all orders as strictly as if they were IV or medication orders.
- ✓ Meals will be taken in bed.
- ✓ Meals will be supervised by a nurse or sitter.
- ✓ Bedside water and decaffeinated herbal tea ad lib (or per fluid restriction 2000 – 3000 mL) unless otherwise indicated.

**Telephone:**
- ✓ No telephone in room.
- ✓ No cell phones in room.
- ✓ Patient will have **no phone privileges** except for one call per day to parents or guardian.

**Visitors:**
- ✓ No visitors except for parents.
- ✓ Parents, nurses, and sitters are to remember that food, fat, diet, weight, and exercise are not appropriate subjects for conversation.

# Legacy Emanuel Children's Hospital
Eating Disorder Hospital Protocol
**Privilege System Phase II**

## Activity:
- ✓ Patients at this phase are on modified medical bedrest and are to remain in bed at all times.
- ✓ Patients may have three 15-minute excursions a day by wheelchair in telemetry range only. **\*You must notify the nurse prior to the excursion.** An adult must go on these excursions and they are to push the wheelchair.
- ✓ The schoolteacher will see you in your room for the first 24 hours. After the first 24 hours, the patient will attend school via wheelchair.
- ✓ Range of motion with Physical Therapy in room.

## Room:
- ✓ Room temperature to be set at 75-80°F at all times.

## Bathroom/Hygiene:
- ✓ Bathroom door will be kept locked.
- ✓ Bathroom privileges are by wheelchair with assistance from the nurse only.
- ✓ Bed bath may be taken with assistance from the nurse.
- ✓ May brush teeth in the bathroom while sitting down.
- ✓ Sweatshirt and long pants to be work when outside of room.

## Meals:
- ✓ Food is regarded as medicine for our purposes. Nursing staff and the patients will follow all orders as strictly as if they were IV or medication orders.
- ✓ Meals will be served when the patient is in bed.
- ✓ Meals will be supervised by a nurse or sitter.
- ✓ Bedside water and decaffeinated herbal tea (provided by the hospital only) ad lib or per fluid restriction (2000-3000 mL).

## Telephone/Internet:
- ✓ No telephone in room.
- ✓ No cell phones in room.
- ✓ Patient will have no phone privileges except for one call per day to parents or guardian if they live out of town.
- ✓ No Internet unless authorized by doctors. To use computer the Wi-Fi card must be removed.

## Visitors:
- ✓ No visitors except for parents.
- ✓ Parents, nurses, and sitters are to remember that food, fat, diet, weight, and exercise are not appropriate subjects for conversation.

# Legacy Emanuel Children's Hospital
Eating Disorder Hospital Protocol
**Privilege System Phase III**

**Activity:**
- ✓ Patients at this phase are on modified ambulatory activity but are to remain in bed except for one of the following:
  - o May sit in the window seat if warmly dressed.
  - o If orthostatic, transport to all activities must be by wheelchair.
  - o If not orthostatic, patients may walk to the dining room, bathroom, classroom, and ordered therapies on the third floor.
- ✓ Patients will go to school every day.
- ✓ Three 15-minute excursions are allowed at this phase. Patients must go in a wheelchair. **\*You must notify the nurse prior to the excursion.** An adult must go on these excursions and they are to push the wheelchair. These excursions may be off the floor unless otherwise indicated.
- ✓ When the patient is off the floor for ordered group therapy, they must go by wheelchair.

**Room:**
- ✓ Room temperature to be set at 75-80°F at all times.

**Bathroom/Hygiene:**
- ✓ Bathroom door will be kept locked.
- ✓ Bathroom privileges are by wheelchair with assistance from the nurse when orthostatic and by foot when not orthostatic.
- ✓ May brush teeth in the bathroom while sitting down.
- ✓ Sweatshirt and long pants to be worn when outside room.

**Meals:**
- ✓ Food is regarded as medicine for our purposes. Nursing staff and the patients will follow all orders as strictly as if they were IV or medication orders.
- ✓ Meals will be in the dining room unless otherwise ordered, always with staff supervision.
- ✓ Meals that are in the room will be in a chair, supervised by a staff member.
- ✓ Bedside water and decaffeinated herbal tea (provided by the hospital only) ad lib or per fluid restriction (2000-3000 mL) unless otherwise indicated.
- ✓ Sugared Gum is allowed. No more than 3 pieces per day. No sugarless gum.

**Telephone/Internet:**
- ✓ No telephone in room.
- ✓ No cell phones in room.
- ✓ Patients will have no phone privileges except for one call per day to parents or guardian if they live out of town.
- ✓ No Internet unless authorized by doctors. To use personal computer the Wi-Fi card must be removed.

**Visitors:**
- ✓ No visitors except for parents. Parents, nurses, and sitters are to remember that food, fat, diet, weight, and exercise are not appropriate subjects for conversation.

# Legacy Emanuel Children's Hospital
### Eating Disorder Hospital Protocol
### Privilege System Phase IV

**Activity:**
- ✓ Patients at this phase are Ambulatory but are to remain in bed whenever orthostatic by blood pressure.
- ✓ If orthostatic by blood pressure, all excursions in and out of room are by wheelchair.
- ✓ If orthostatic by heart rate only and daytime heart rate is equal to or greater than 50 beats per minute, patient may walk **with accompaniment** to school, group, meals, bathroom, excursions, and therapies within the hospital.
- ✓ Three 15-minute excursions are allowed at this phase with an adult. **\*You must notify the nurse prior to the excursion.** Excursions may be off the floor.
- ✓ When the patient is walking on excursions, they must use the elevator. Our patients are never to use the stairs except in case of fire.
- ✓ School is mandatory for all patients who have not graduated from high school.
- ✓ When not orthostatic, patients may spend as much time as they like in the activity room. A parent and/or staff must supervise patients. The patient must mainly be sitting during activities.

**Room:**
- ✓ Room temperature to be set at 75-80°F at all times.

**Bathroom/Hygiene:**
- ✓ Bathroom door will be kept locked.
- ✓ Bathroom privileges may be on foot with assistance from nurse, when not orthostatic.
- ✓ Bathroom privileges will be by wheelchair when orthostatic by blood pressure.
- ✓ Patient may take a shower while standing when not orthostatic by blood pressure, in the shower chair with assistance when orthostatic by blood pressure. Showers will continue to be observed by nurse or parent.
- ✓ May brush teeth standing when not orthostatic by blood pressure, and sitting when orthostatic by blood pressure.
- ✓ Sweatshirt and long pants to be worn when outside of room.

**Meals:**
- ✓ Food is regarded as medicine for our purposes, and nursing staff and the patients will follow all orders as strictly as if they were IV or medication orders.
- ✓ Meals will be in the dining room unless otherwise ordered, always with staff supervision.
- ✓ Meals that are in the room will be out of bed and in a chair, supervised by a staff member.
- ✓ Bedside water and decaffeinated herbal tea (provided by the hospital only) ad lib or per fluid restriction (2000-3000 mL) unless otherwise indicated.
- ✓ Sugared gum is allowed. No more than 3 pieces per day. No sugarless gum.

**Telephone/Internet:**
- ✓ No telephone in room.
- ✓ No cell phone in room.
- ✓ Patient will have no phone privileges except for one call a day to parents or guardian if they live out of town.
- ✓ No Internet unless authorized by doctors. To use personal computer the Wi-Fi card must be removed.

**Visitors:**
- ✓ No visitors except for parents.
- ✓ Parents, nurses, and sitters are to remember that food, fat, diet, weight, and exercise are not appropriate subjects for conversation.

# Appendix D

**LECH Pediatric In-Patient**
**Eating Disorder Admission Orders**

ALL LISTED ORDERS ARE IN EFFECT UNLESS CROSSED OUT. **EXCEPTIONS:** ORDERS PRECEDED BY A BOX
(☐) REQUIRE A (✓) TO INITIATE. ORDERS WITH BLANKS INDICATE ADDITIONALLY INFORMATION IS NEEDED.

| DATE: | TIME: | HEIGHT: | WEIGHT: | ALLERGIES: |
|---|---|---|---|---|
| | | | | |

1. Admit to Pediatrics. Attending:_____
2. Primary Care Physician:_____
3. Diagnosis:_____
4. Phase: ☐ I ☐ II ☐ III ☐ IV
5. Diet:
   - ☐ Starting Calories/Day (full fat diet) ☐ 800 ☐ 1000 ☐ 1200 ☐ 1500 ☐ 2000 ☐ 2150 ÷ 3 meals
     - ☐ Other_____ and one afternoon snack.
   - ☐ Vegetarian choices only (full fat diet).
   - ☐ Give all calories as food.
   - ☐ Give calories as 1.5cal/mL liquid supplement ever y 4 hours (order no food).
   - ☐ 50% of calories to be given in the form of 1.5 cal/mL liquid supplement and 50% as food the first day; 75% as food and 25% supplement the second day and 100% as food thereafter if tolerated by patient.
   - ☐ Give one can of 1.5 cal/mL liquid supplement at bedtime.
   - ☐ Do not force food consumption. If patient is unable to eat all the food, RN is to substitute 1.5cal/mL of liquid supplement calorie for calorie.
   - ☐ If patient refuses to drink supplement to meet caloric requirement, give via NG tube. Notify attending, not H.O. for NG orders.
   - ☐ If patient admitted too late for a tray, substitute 1 can 1.5 cal/mL liquid supplement.
6. Notify case manager of admission.
7. Call H.O. when patient arrives on floor.
8. Nutritionist to figure retrospective calories daily.
9. Vitals are to be completed by RN or LPN. Do not leave room during the measurement of vital signs. Orthostatic vitals are obtained by having the patient lie for 5 minutes, taking BP and apical heart rate then having the patient stand for two minutes and repeat BO and apical heart rate.
10. Vitals:
    a. 2300-0600: Non orthostatic pulse, temperature, respirations and assessments Q 4 H.
    b. 0600-2200: Orthostatic vital signs, temperature, respirations and assessments Q 4 H X 48 H.
    c. 0600-2200: If HR less than or equal to 40 BPM before vitals, hold orthostatic vital signs, do regular vital signs, temperature, respirations, and assessments. ☐ Q 4 H ☐ Q 6 H ☐ Q 12 H
11. Please note and flag in comment on computer the following conditions:
    Postural change: decrease in systolic BP greater than or equal to 10 mm Hg when standing.
    Postural change: increased pulse greater than or equal to 35 BPM when standing.
    Pulse: less than or equal to 45 BPM.
    Temperature less than 36.3°C (days and evenings); less than 36°C (nights)
12. Temperature instability:
    Bair Hugger Blanket if Temp less than 36.3°C (days) or less than 36°C (nights).
13. For pulse less than 40 BPM first check temperature. If temp less than 36.3°C days or evenings or less than 36°C at night, place Bair Hugger Blanket. If already on, turn the blanket up. Recheck Q 30 minutes until temperature is stable. If pulse less than 40 BPM and temperature is stable give one can of 1 cal/mL liquid supplement. If heart rate consistently between 30-40 BPM, may lower telemetry limit to 30 BPM. Do not give more supplement. If H less than 30 BPM consistently, notify HO to physically check patient for level of consciousness when awakened and then notify attending and document. Check BP (resting).

**Order NOTED (name/date/time)** _____ **Order PROCESSED (name/date/time)** _____

Physician/Credentialed Provider's Signature: _____

Printed Name: _____ Provider #: _____
**All Pre- Printed Orders must have a Physician/Credentialed Provider's signature to initiate.**

| ALL LISTED ORDERS ARE IN EFFECT UNLESS CROSSED OUT. **EXCEPTIONS:** ORDERS PRECEDED BY A BOX (□) REQUIRE A (✓) TO INITIATE. ORDERS WITH BLANKS INDICATE ADDITIONALLY INFORMATION IS NEEDED. |
|---|

| DATE: | TIME: | HEIGHT: | WEIGHT: | ALLERGIES: |
|---|---|---|---|---|

14. Daily weight before 8:30 AM after void, in hospital gown only (no underwear, jewelry, or telemetry box), before any PO intake. Chart in computer and on graphic sheet.
15. Strict Intake and Output. Specific gravity Q void, for 1st 24 H, then once a shift. Daily fluid total 2000 mL/day minimum and 3000 mL/day maximum.
16. Strict Calorie counts. (Chart in computer when available).
17. EKG on admission.
18. Telemetry: No pulse oximetry check please.
    - □ Limit settings: Upper limit: 140 BPM       Lower limit: 45 BPM.
    - □ By 6:30 AM each day, place lowest Heart Rate Strip in chart.
19. Labs:
    - □ CBC
    - □ Sed Rate
    - □ Comprehensive panel
    - □ TSH, Free T4
    - □ FSH, LH, if female
    - □ Estradiol, if female (send out if needed for exact quantitative level)
    - □ HCG (qualitative), if female.
    - □ Expanded urine drug screen (with first void on admission)
    - □ Phosphorus Q 6 hours times 24 hours, then daily thereafter
    - □ Metabolic cart study
    - □ Testosterone levels, if male
    - □ Dexascan of lumbar spine (indication: weight loss)
    - □ Insulin level
    - □ ASO titer
    - □ Throat culture
    - □ Anti DNASE-B
    - □ Leptin Level (Please send to Labcorp)
    _____
20. Place IV Heparin lock.
21. Medications:
    - □ Zinc Sulfate 110mg PO Q AM (maximum 4 mg/kg/day)
    - □ Calcium Carbonate 500 mg (Tums®) 1 tab PO b.i.d.
    - □ Adult Multivitamin 1 tablet PO Q AM for patients 11 years of age and older (maximum dose 2 tablets daily).
    - □ Children's chewable multivitamin 1 tablet PO Q AM for patients younger than 11 years of age (maximum dose 2 tablets daily).
    - □ Heparin 10 units/1 mL IV flush Q 8 H and p.r.n. (not to exceed 50 units/kg/day).
    - □ Anesthetic cream applied topically 30 minutes prior to IV start and venipuncture.
22. Lock on bathroom door.
23. □ Sitter.
24. Consults: Child life, pet therapy, art therapy, physical therapy, and occupational therapy.
    - □ Cardiology
    - □ CRC (social services)
    - □ _____
25. Obtain consent for group therapy attendance.

**Order NOTED (name/date/time)** _____ **Order PROCESSED (name/date/time)** _____

Physician/Credentialed Provider's Signature: _____

Printed Name: _____ Provider #: _____
**All Pre- Printed Orders must have a Physician/Credentialed Provider's signature to initiate.**

# Index

AAP guidelines, 157
    anorexia nervosa, 157
    bulimia nervosa, 157
Addison's disease, 49
amenorrhea, 44, 59, 85, 116, 263
AN subtypes, 60
    purging anorexia, 61
    restricting anorexia, 60
anemia, 46
anorexia nervosa, 3–6
    purger, 62
    restrictor, 62
anorexogenic families, 17, 234
antipsychotics, 94, 127, 132
anxiety, 42, 43, 99, 123–195
    anxiety disorder, 179, 254, 268

biopsychosocial approach, 137
BMI, 47, 190, 248
bradycardia, 41, 79, 87, 151, 156, 157, 176, 197
brain tumors, 48
bulimia nervosa, 15, 63, 95–97, 102, 209

caffiene, 41, 42, 159, 189, 197
cardiologist, 79–88, 161
carotenemia, 45
cholesterol, 18, 190
cognitive deficits, 48
constipation, 85, 88, 205
consumptive disease, 9
cooking, 39, 175, 210, 229, 235
CT scan, 49, 191, 275

daughter, 78, 150, 218, 220, 242
Day Treatment Unit (DTU), 60, 153, 193, 272, 278
denial, 47
depression, 80, 123–125, 146, 275
DEXA (bone densitometry), 176, 190, 233
Diagnostic and Statistical manual of Mental disorders (DSM), 53–57
diarrhea, 85
diet pills, 35, 42, 50, 189
dietician, 104, 230, 236, 239
drug abuse, 62, 72, 200

alchohol, 62, 72

drug and alchohol evaluation, 238

urine drug screening, 189

dysphagia, 54, 56, 67, 265, 266

EDNOS, 53–94

electrolytes, 46, 86, 186, 188

endocrinologist, 85–88

gastro-endocrinologist, 88

Pediatric Endocrinologist, 49

enzymes, 46, 86, 189

estradiol level, 44, 86, 189

exercise, 37, 51, 203, 261

exercise restriction, 177

family practitioner, 80, 161, 216

famine, 39, 110–116

father, 61–64, 82, 104, 262, 274–276

feminist theory, 16

figures

bone density scan, 249

growth chart of "Bob", 253

growth chart of "Myron", 252

stress v. genetic load, 103

tanner stages, 32

The Kartini clinic meal plan (KCMP), 226

food hoarding, 35, 50

food phobia, 54, 67, 128–129, 265–278

gay, 234, 258

grandfather, 251

grandmother, 51, 100

grocery shopping, 195, 208, 210, 232

growth hormone studies, 86

gynecologist, 44

heritability, 99–106, 139

hormones, 44, 85, 116, 241, 246, 250

hormone replacement, 190

hospital, 2–7, 21–27, 42–43, 67–83, 151–188

Legacy Emanuel Children's Hospital, 176, 194

hypokalemia, 79, 156, 186, 276

hypomagnesaemia, 188

hyponatremia, 40, 276

hypophosphatemia, 79, 168, 186–188

hypothermia, 43, 158

hypothyroidism, 84, 85, 116

Ideal body weight (IBW), 32, 161–165, 246
  determining, 162
insomnia, 85, 205, 238, 241
ipecac, 50

karyotype, 86, 87

lactose intolerance, 36
laxatives, 35, 47, 50, 134, 188

media, 18, 30, 76, 174
medical instability, 79–83, 159, 188, 198
medication, 121–136, 191–195, 238, 269–276
  herbal, 10, 134
mental illness, 50, 200, 211, 261
milieu, 60, 196, 201, 207–208
  homogenous milieu, 199
  milieu therapist, 178, 198, 202, 204, 207, 209, 278
Minnesota semi-starvation study (MSSS), 109–119
  bones, 116
  fat mass, 115
  heart size in children, 115
  increased relative hydration, 116
  pituitary gland, 116
  psychological consequences, 117
  skeletal muscle mass, 115
  thyroid gland, 116
mood instability, 40, 51
mother, 71, 104, 247, 254, 262
MRI, 49, 86, 87, 91, 191, 275
munchhausen by proxy, 49

narcissism, 12
naso-gastric feeds, 269
neoroimaging, 95–98
neutropenia, 46
nutritionist, 7, 236, 239, 262

obsessive compulsive disorder (OCD), 123, 179, 189, 195, 254
olanzapine, 127, 132, 269, 273–275, 278
oral contraceptive, 44, 190
orthostasis, 43, 79–83, 151, 160, 197, 198

PANDAS (pediatric autoimmune neuropsychiatric disorders associated with streptococcus), 189
pediatrician, 2, 27, 30–36, 83–86, 147, 202, 233

polyuria, 110

Portland, Oregon, 1, 6, 78, 174, 180, 194, 276

pregnancy, 59, 85

pregnancy test, 189

professional anorexics, 262

psychiatrist, 1–20, 71, 77, 93, 205

psychoanalysis, 4, 11

psychogenic drinking, 40, 51

psychogenic polydipsia, 116

psychologist, 246, 266, 274, 277

psychopharmacology, 94, 121, 125, 239

quetiapine, 127

re-feeding, 119, 151, 181

REDS-Child (rating of eating disorder severity), 46–49, 148

interview, 148, 150

relapse, 198, 216–222, 243, 273

remission, 174, 215–223, 240–243

restaurant, 65, 208, 210

risperidone, 127

Russell's sign, 45, 147

schizophrenia, 9, 93, 97, 200

sedimentation rate (ESR), 188

seizures, 40

sex, 60, 149

sex abuse, 15, 258

sexual drive, 76, 119

STD, 19

social withdrawal, 33, 38, 51, 217

son, 10, 82, 150, 220, 258, 274

sports, 21, 75, 204, 240, 261

SSRI (selective serotonin re-uptake inhibitor), 41, 55, 63, 125–127, 132, 268

swollen glands, 46

syncope (fainting), 34, 49, 151, 167

pre-syncope, 34

tanner stages (SMR), 32, 58, 154, 256

teenagers, 19–34, 228

The Kartini clinic meal plan (KCMP), 223, 224, 227, 232–233

The Kartini inpatient eating-disorder unit, 170

thelarche, 31

therapy, 246

art, 59, 178, 205

family, 66, 135, 209, 234

group, 64, 135, 178, 202, 209, 237

hypnotherapy, 206, 238

individual, 205, 209, 238, 247

massage, 205

occupational (OT), 178, 204

parent, 175

pet, 238

physical (PT), 178, 203, 210

  yoga, 204, 210

thyroid, 85–86

thyroid gland, 116

thyroid studies, 189

tooth erosion, 45

violent behavior, 99

vomitus, 35, 51, 92

young adults, 139, 208–212, 219, 234